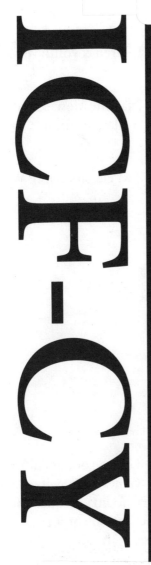

ICF-CY

International Classification of Functioning, Disability and Health

Children & Youth Version

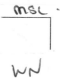
BIRMINGHAM City University

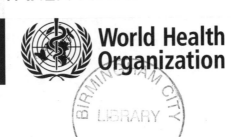 **World Health Organization**

WHO Library Cataloguing-in-Publication Data

International classification of functioning, disability and health : children & youth version : ICF-CY.

1.Child development - classification. 2.Adolescent development - classification. 3.Body constitution. 4.Disability evaluation. 5.Health status. 6.Causality. 7.Classification. 8.Manuals I.World Health Organization. II.Title: ICF-CY.

ISBN **978 92 4 154732 1**   (NLM classification: W 15)

Typeset in India
Printed in India

Contents

ICF-CY Preface   v

ICF-CY Introduction   ix
    1. Background   xi
    2. Purpose of the ICF-CY   xii
    3. Development of the ICF-CY   xiii
    4. Information for ICF-CY users   xviii
    5. Case vignettes   xxii
    6. Acknowledgements   xxv

ICF Introduction   1
    1. Background   3
    2. Aims of ICF   5
    3. Properties of ICF   7
    4. Overview of ICF components   9
    5. Model of Functioning and Disability   17
    6. Use of ICF   20

ICF-CY One-level classification   25

ICF-CY Two-level classification   29

ICF-CY Detailed classification with definitions   43
    Body Functions   45
    Body Structures   107
    Activities and Participation   129
    Environmental Factors   189

ICF Annexes   225
    1. Taxonomic and terminological issues   227
    2. Guidelines for coding ICF   234
    3. Possible uses of the Activities and Participation list   248
    4. Case examples   252
    5. ICF and people with disabilities   255
    6. Ethical guidelines for the use of ICF   257
    7. Summary of the revision process   259
    8. Future directions for the ICF   263

9. Suggested ICF data requirements for ideal and minimal health information systems or surveys 265

10. Acknowledgements 266

ICF-CY Index to Introductions and Annexes 281

ICF-CY Index to categories within classifications 289

ICF-CY

Preface

The first two decades of life are characterized by rapid growth and significant changes in the physical, social and psychological development of children and youth. Parallel changes define the nature and complexity of children's environments across infancy, early childhood, middle childhood and adolescence. Each of these changes is associated with their growing competence, societal participation and independence.

The *International Classification of Functioning, Disability and Health for Children and Youth (ICF-CY)* is derived from the *International Classification of Functioning, Disability and Health* (ICF) (WHO, 2001) and is designed to record the characteristics of the developing child and the influence of its surrounding environment.

The ICF-CY can be used by providers, consumers and all those concerned with the health, education, and well-being of children and youth. It provides a common and universal language for clinical, public health and research applications to facilitate the documentation and measurement of health and disability in children and youth.

The classification builds on the ICF conceptual framework and uses a common language and terminology for recording problems involving functions and structures of the body, activity limitations and participation restrictions manifested in infancy, childhood and adolescence and relevant environmental factors.

The ICF-CY belongs to the "family" of international classifications developed by WHO for application to various aspects of health. The WHO Family of International Classifications (WHO-FIC) provides a framework to code a wide range of information about health (e.g. diagnosis, functioning and disability, and reasons for contact with health services), and uses a standardized language permitting communication about health and health care across the world in various disciplines and sciences. In WHO's international classifications, health conditions, such as diseases, disorders and injuries are classified primarily in ICD-10, which provides an etiological framework. Functioning and disability associated with health conditions are classified in ICF. These two classifications are complementary and should be used together. The ICF-CY can assist clinicians, educators, researchers, administrators, policy-makers and parents to document the characteristics of children and youth that are of importance in promoting their growth, health and development.

The ICF-CY was developed in response to a need for a version of the ICF that could be used universally for children and youth in the health, education and social sectors. The manifestations of disability and health conditions in children and adolescents are different in nature, intensity and impact from those of adults. These differences need to be taken into account so that classification content is sensitive to the changes associated with development and encompasses the characteristics of different age groups and environments.

Between 2002 and 2005, a WHO Work Group[1] for ICF-CY held a series of meetings[2] and field trials to review existing ICF codes and identify new codes to describe the characteristics of children and youth. This publication is the outcome of that process[3] and includes dimensions, classes and codes to document body functions and structures, activities and participation of children and youth, and their environments across developmental stages. Drawing on the guidelines in Annex 8 of the ICF, the version for children and youth is consistent with the organization and structure of the main volume.

Development activities took the form of:

(a) modifying or expanding descriptions;

(b) assigning new content to unused codes;

(c) modifying inclusion and exclusion criteria; and

(d) expanding qualifiers to include developmental aspects.

Thus, this derived version of the ICF for children and youth expands the coverage of the main ICF volume by providing specific content and additional detail to more fully cover the body functions and structures, activities and participation, and environments of particular relevance to infants, toddlers, children and adolescents.[4] With its functional emphasis, the ICF-CY uses a common language that can be applied across disciplines as well as national boundaries to advance services, policy and research on behalf of children and youth.

---

[1] Core members of the work group were Eva Bjorck-Akesson of Sweden, Judith Hollenweger (Switzerland), Don Lollar (the United States of America), Andrea Martinuzzi (Italy) and Huib Ten Napel (the Netherlands) with Matilde Leonardi (Italy) and Rune J. Simeonsson (USA) serving as co-chair and chair, respectively. In WHO, Nenad Kostanjsek managed and coordinated the efforts of the ICF-CY work group under the overall guidance of T. Bedirhan Üstün. Primary financial support of work group activities was provided by the National Center on Birth Defects and Developmental Disabilities of the Centers for Disease Control and Prevention (CDC), USA. Additional support was provided by national ministries in Italy and Sweden, the United Nations Educational, Scientific and Cultural Organization, WHO and universities of respective work group members.

[2] The first was a meeting in conjunction with the official introduction of the ICF by WHO to health ministers of the world at Trieste, Italy, in the spring of 2002. Subsequent meetings between 2002 and 2005 involved working sessions in various countries with local participation by representatives of consumer, service, policy and research communities.

[3] A first draft version of the ICF-CY was produced in 2003 and field tested in 2004. Subsequently, the beta draft of the ICF-CY was developed and field tested in 2005. A pre-final version of the ICF-CY was submitted to WHO at the end of 2005 for expert review. Recommendations from that review process were incorporated into the final version submitted at the annual meeting of the Network of WHO Collaborating Centres for the Family of International Classifications (WHO-FIC) in Tunis in the autumn of 2006. The ICF-CY was officially accepted for publication as the first derived classification of the ICF in November 2006.

[4] Although the addition of new codes and modification of existing codes in the ICF-CY were made specifically for children and youth, they may also be relevant to the ICF. Hence, the new or modified codes in ICF-CY have been incorporated into the ICF updating process.

ICF-CY

Introduction

1. Background

This volume contains the *International Classification of Functioning, Disability and Health for Children and Youth and is* known as the ICF-CY. The ICF-CY is derived from, and compatible with, the *International Classification of Functioning, Disability and Health* (ICF) (WHO, 2001). As such, it includes further detailed information on the application of the ICF when documenting the characteristics of children and youth below the age of 18 years. The original introduction and annexes of the ICF have been incorporated into this volume.

As a derived classification, the ICF-CY was prepared by "adopting the reference classification structure and categories, providing additional detail beyond that provided by the reference classification" (WHO-FIC, 2004, p. 5). Drawing on the guidelines in Annex 8 of the ICF, the ICF-CY was designed to be compatible with the organization and structure of the main volume.

Development activities took the form of:

(a) modifying or expanding descriptions;

(b) assigning new content to unused codes;

(c) modifying inclusion and exclusion criteria; and

(d) expanding qualifiers to encompass developmental aspects.[5]

Thus, the ICF-CY expands the coverage of the main volume through the addition of content and greater detail to encompass the body functions and structures, activities, participation and environments specific to infants, toddlers, children and adolescents.

The age range covered by the ICF-CY is from birth to 18 years of age, paralleling the age range of other United Nations conventions (e.g. UN Convention on the Rights of the Child, 1989). As a member of the WHO Family of International Classifications (WHO-FIC), the ICF-CY complements the ICD-10, and other derived and related classifications, by providing a framework and standard language for the description of health and health-related states in children and youth.

---

[5] Although the addition of new codes and modification of existing codes in the ICF-CY were made with particular relevance to children and youth, they may also be relevant to the ICF. Hence, the new or modified codes in ICF-CY have been incorporated into the ICF update process.

2. Purpose of the ICF-CY

The ICF-CY is intended for use by clinicians, educators, policy-makers, family members, consumers and researchers to document characteristics of health and functioning in children and youth. The ICF-CY offers a conceptual framework and a common language and terminology for recording problems manifested in infancy, childhood and adolescence involving functions and structures of the body, activity limitations and participation restrictions, and environmental factors important for children and youth. With its emphasis on functioning, the ICF-CY can be used across disciplines, government sectors and national boundaries to define and document the health, functioning and development of children and youth.

3. Development of the ICF-CY

The development of the ICF-CY is summarized in terms of:

(a) the practical and philosophical rationales for its elaboration; and

(b) key issues informing the process.

A brief history of development activities is given in the preface.

3.1 Rationale for the ICF-CY

The rationale for the development of the ICF-CY was based on practical, philosophical, taxonomic and public health considerations.

A. Practical rationale

From a practical perspective, the need for a comprehensive classification of childhood disability that could be used across service systems has been recognized for some time, but not realized. Moreover, the implementation of children's rights in the form of access to health care, education, and social and habilitation services required a classification system sensitive to the physical, social and psychological characteristics unique to children and youth. Thus, the ICF-CY was developed to capture the universe of functioning in children and youth. Further, the manifestations of functioning, disability and health conditions in childhood and adolescence are different in nature, intensity and impact from those of adults. These differences were taken into account and the ICF-CY was developed in a manner sensitive to changes associated with growth and development.

B. Philosophical rationale

From a philosophical perspective, it was essential that a classification defining the health and functioning of children and youth incorporate the fundamental human rights defined by the UN Convention on the Rights of Persons with Disabilities (UN, 2007). As a taxonomy derived from the ICF, the ICF-CY describes states of functioning and health in codes with greater granularity which serve as precursors of more mature functioning. The rationale for a public health framework was based on the promise of a population approach to preventing disability in childhood. All content in the ICF-CY is in conformity with international conventions and declarations on behalf of the rights of children. Hence, the documentation of categories and codes in the ICF-CY may serve as evidence in assuring the rights of children and youth.

The major themes of these conventions and declarations are summarized below, with emphasis on the most vulnerable children and youth – those with disabilities.

1989 UN Convention on the Rights of the Child with particular reference to article 23

"A mentally or physically disabled child should enjoy a full and decent life in conditions which ensure dignity, promotes self reliance and facilitates the child's active participation in the community" (Article 23(1)).

This article of the Convention specifies that children with disabilities have the right to special care with assistance provided to children and caregivers appropriate to the child's condition. Assistance is to be provided free-of-charge and designed to provide effective access to education, training, health-care and rehabilitation services in order to promote the child's social integration and individual development.

Standard Rules for the Equalization of Opportunities (1994)

Rule 6 recognizes the principle of equal primary, secondary and tertiary educational opportunities for children, youth and adults with disabilities in integrated settings. Further, it emphasizes the importance of early intervention and special attention for very young children and preschool children with disabilities.

Education for all: The World Education Forum in Dakar (2000)

The Forum advocated for the expansion of early childhood care and education, and the provision of free and compulsory education for all. Additional goals include promoting learning and skills for young people and adults, increasing adult literacy, achieving gender parity and gender equality, and enhancing educational quality.

Salamanca Statement on the Right to Education (2001)

The Salamanca Statement declares that every child has a fundamental right to education and that special educational needs arise from disabilities or learning difficulties. The Statement also asserts that all children should be accommodated with child-centred pedagogy. In addition, the Statement emphasizes access to regular schooling with inclusive orientation for children with disabilities and the importance of early education to promote development and school-readiness.

UN Convention on the Rights of Persons with Disabilities (2006)

"[…] Children with disabilities should have full enjoyment of all human rights and fundamental freedoms on an equal basis with other children, and recalling obligations to that end undertaken by States Parties to the Convention on the Rights of the Child […]" (Preamble).

"1. States Parties shall take all necessary measures to ensure the full enjoyment by children with disabilities of all human rights and fundamental freedoms on an equal basis with other children. 2. In all actions concerning children with disabilities, the best interests of the child shall be a primary consideration. 3. States Parties shall ensure that children with disabilities have the right to express their views freely on all matters affecting them, their views being given due weight in accordance with their age and maturity, on an equal basis with other children, and to be provided with disability and age-appropriate assistance to realize that right" (Article 7).

Article 30 of the Convention focuses on participation on an equal basis with others and underlines the importance for children with disabilities to play, participate in sports activities and cultural life. "Participation in cultural life, recreation, leisure and sport: 1. States Parties recognize the right of persons with disabilities to take part on an equal basis with others in cultural life […] to have the opportunity to develop and utilize their creative, artistic and intellectual potential, not only for their own benefit, but also for the enrichment of society; [...] to ensure that laws protecting intellectual property rights do not constitute an unreasonable or discriminatory barrier to access by persons with disabilities to cultural materials [...] to recognition and support of their specific cultural and linguistic identity, including sign languages and deaf culture. [...] to participate on an equal basis with others in recreational, leisure and sporting activities [...], children with disabilities have equal access with other children to participate in play, recreation and leisure, and sporting activities, including those activities in the school system;" (Article 30).

3.2   Issues relating to children and youth in the ICF-CY

Children's growth and development constitute central themes guiding the identification and adaptation of the content for the ICF-CY. Many issues informed the addition or expansion of content, including the nature of cognition and language, play, disposition and behaviour in the developing child. Particular attention was given to four key issues in the derivation of the ICF-CY.

The child in the context of the family

Development is a dynamic process by which the child moves progressively from dependency on others for all activities in infancy towards physical, social and psychological maturity and independence in adolescence. In this dynamic process, the child's functioning is dependent on continuous interactions with the family or other caregivers in a close, social environment. Therefore, the functioning of the child cannot be seen in isolation but rather in terms of the child in the context of the family system. This is an important consideration in making judgements about the child's functioning in life situations. The influence of family interactions on the child's functioning is greater in this developmental phase than at any later point in an individual's lifespan. Further, as these interactions frame the acquisition of various skills over the first two decades of life, the role of the physical and social environment is crucial.

Developmental delay

In children and youth, there are variations in the time of emergence of body functions, structures and the acquisition of skills associated with individual differences in growth and development. Lags in the emergence of functions, structures or capacities may not be permanent but reflect delayed development. They are manifested in each domain (e.g. cognitive functions, speech functions, mobility and communication), are age-specific and are influenced by physical as well as psychological factors in the environment.

These variations in the emergence of body functions, structures or performance of expected developmental skills define the concept of developmental delay and often serve as the basis for identifying children with an increased risk of disabilities. An important consideration in the development of the ICF-CY pertained to the nature of the qualifier used to document the severity or magnitude of a problem of Body Functions, Body Structures, and Activities and Participation. In the main volume of the ICF, the universal severity qualifier for all domains encompasses five levels from (0) no impairment, difficulty or barrier to (4) complete impairment, difficulty or barrier. With children, it is important to consider the concept of a lag or delay in the emergence of functions, structures, activities and participation in the assignment of a severity qualifier. The ICF-CY includes, therefore, the term and concept of delay to define the universal qualifier for Body Functions and Structure, and Activities and Participation. This allows for documentation of the extent or magnitude of lags or delays in the emergence of functions, structures and capacity, and in the performance of activities and participation in a child, recognizing that the severity of the qualifier codes may change over time.

Participation

Participation is defined as a person's "involvement in a life situation" and represents the societal perspective of functioning. As the nature and settings of life situations of children and youth differ significantly from those of adults, participation has received special attention in the ICF-CY. With development, life situations change dramatically in number and complexity from the relationship with a primary caregiver and solitary play of the very young child to social play, peer relationships and schooling of children at later ages. The younger the child, the more likely it is that opportunities to participate are defined by parents, caregivers or service providers. The role of the family environment and others in the immediate environment is integral to understanding participation, especially in early childhood.

The ability to be engaged and interact socially develops in the young child's close relations with others, such as parents, siblings and peers in its immediate environment. The social environment remains significant as a factor throughout the period of development but the nature and complexity of the environment changes from early childhood through to adolescence.

Environments

Environmental factors are defined as "the physical, social and attitudinal environment in which people live and conduct their lives". The person-environment interaction implicit in the paradigm shift from a medical to a broader biopsychosocial model of disability requires special attention to environmental factors for children and youth. A central issue is that the nature and complexity of children's environments change dramatically with transitions across the stages of infancy, early childhood, middle childhood and adolescence. Changes in the environments of children and youth are associated with their increasing competence and independence.

The environments of children and youth can be viewed in terms of a series of successive systems surrounding them from the most immediate to the most distant, each differing in its influence as a function of the age or stage of the developing child. The restricted environments of the infant and young child reflect their limited mobility and the need to assure their safety and security. The young child is significantly dependent on persons in the immediate environment. Products for personal use must be adapted to the child's developmental level. Objects for play and access to peers, for example, are essential components of major life situations of young children. For older children, the environments of their everyday life are closely connected to home and school and, for youth, gradually become more diversified into environments in the larger context of community and society.

Given the dependence of the developing child, the physical and social elements of the environment have a significant impact on its functioning. Negative environmental factors often have a stronger impact on children than on adults. A child's lack of nutritious food, access to clean water, and a safe and sanitary setting, for example, not only contributes to disease and compromises health but also impairs its functioning and ability to learn. Thus, intervention and prevention efforts to promote children's health and well-being focus on modification or enhancement of the physical, social or psychological environment.

Alteration of the physical environment immediate to the child involves the provision of food, shelter and safety. The provision of assistive devices or technology represents environmental alterations that may facilitate functioning in a child with significant physical impairments.

Alteration of the social and psychological elements of the child's immediate environment may involve social support for the family and education for caregivers.

The nature and extent of environmental support will vary according to the age of the child with the needs of the young child differing from those of an infant or adolescent. Alterations in environments less immediate to children may take the form of legislation or national policies to ensure their access to health care, social services and education.

4. Information for ICF-CY users

4.1 Uses of the ICF-CY

The ICF-CY defines components of health and health-related components of well-being. Among children and youth these components include mental functions of attention, memory and perception as well as activities involving play, learning, family life and education in different domains. The domains of the ICF-CY are defined by two umbrella terms. "Functioning" is a term encompassing all body functions, activities and participation. "Disability" is a term encompassing impairments, activity limitations and participation restrictions. Environmental factors define barriers or facilitators to functioning.

The ICF-CY is using an alphanumeric coding system. The letters "b" for Body Function, "s" for Body Structures, "d" for Activities/Participation and "e" for Environmental Factors are followed by a numeric code that starts with the chapter number (one digit), followed by the second level heading (two digits), and the third and fourth level headings (one digit each). The universal qualifier with values from 0=no problem to 4=complete problem, is entered after the decimal point to specify the extent to which a function or activity differs from an expected or typical state. The negative aspects of environments are qualified in terms of barriers whereas positive values of the universal qualifier are used to denote the facilitating role of environments.[6]

The information provided by the ICF-CY may be used in a variety of ways including in clinical, administrative, surveillance, policy or research applications. In each case, ICF-CY classes can be used to record a single problem or a profile defining a child's health and functioning difficulties.

In clinical applications, ICF-CY classes can provide a summary of assessment findings, clarifying diagnostic information and serving as the basis for planned interventions.

Administratively, information pertaining to eligibility, service provision, reimbursement and follow-up can be recorded with ICF-CY codes. In surveillance applications, a limited set of ICF-CY classes may be selected to standardize data collection procedures across instruments and over time in order to document prevalence of conditions, project service needs and service utilization patterns.

When applied to policy, the conceptual framework of the ICF-CY may be used to frame a particular policy focus, for example, children's right to education.

In research, selected ICF-CY classes may be used to standardize the characteristics of participants, the selection of assessment measures and the definition of outcomes.

In all uses of the ICF-CY, parents, children and youth should be included whenever possible.

---

[6] Detailed information on the coding structure is provided in Annex 2. Guidelines for coding ICF.

4.2 Steps in using the ICF-CY

The classification and coding of dimensions of disability in children and youth is a complex activity requiring consideration of significant limitations of body functions, body structures, activities and participation in physical, social and psychological development. General coding guidelines are presented in Annex 2 of this volume and provide information on the process of assigning codes for health and health-related states. It is highly recommended that users review these guidelines and obtain training in the use of the ICF-CY prior to initiating classification activities. Accurate coding of disability in children and youth requires knowledge of changes in functioning associated with growth and development, as well as the ability to distinguish between developmental changes that are within the normal range and changes that are atypical. Change in functioning is part of the "typical functioning" of a child. It is important, therefore, to recognize that "normality" is age-dependent and implies an understanding of "normal functioning" at a given time and its mediating role on the environments of children and youth.

The unit of classification in the ICF-CY is not a diagnosis for a child, but a profile of its functioning. The purpose of the ICF-CY is to describe the nature and severity of the limitations of the child's functioning and identify the environmental factors influencing such functioning. Although coding may be carried out for a variety of purposes (according to the ethical guidelines in Annex 6), a consistent approach should be followed in order to produce reliable and valid data. When using the ICF-CY, it is mandatory to assign codes based on primary information in the form of direct measurement, observation, first-hand interview and/or professional judgement. It is recognized that the intended use of the ICF-CY is to define the level of detail in coding, which will range from clinical settings to survey applications. The following steps aim to guide users in assigning ICF-CY classes and codes related to problems in children and youth.

(1) Define the information available for coding and identify whether it relates to the domain of Body Functions, Body Structures, Activities/Participation or Environmental Factors.

(2) Locate the chapter (4-character code) within the appropriate domain that most closely corresponds to the information to be coded.

(3) Read the description of the 4-character code and attend to any notes related to the description.

(4) Review any inclusion or exclusion notes that apply to the code and proceed accordingly.

(5) Determine if the information to be coded is consistent with the 4-character level or if a more detailed description at the 5- or 6-character code should be examined.

(6) Proceed to the level of code that most closely corresponds to the information to be coded. Review the description and any inclusion or exclusion notes that apply to the code.

(7) Select the code and review the available information in order to assign a value for the universal qualifier that defines the extent of the impairment in body function and structure, activity limitation, participation restriction (0=no

impairment/difficulty to 4=complete impairment/difficulty) or environmental barrier (0=no barrier to 4=complete barrier) or facilitator (0=no facilitator to +4=complete facilitator).

(8) Assign the code with the qualifier at the 2nd, 3rd or 4th item level. For example, d115.2 (moderate difficulty in listening).

(9) Repeat steps 1 to 8 for each manifestation of function or disability of interest for coding where information is available.

(10) Parents and consumers may participate in the process by completing age-appropriate inventories that allow specific areas of functional concern to be highlighted, but they should do so before full evaluations and codes are provided by professionals or a team of professionals.

4.3 Conventions

The main conventions for this classification are described in the Introduction and Annexes to the ICF, which follows this Introduction to the ICF-CY. They should be read carefully prior to using the ICF-CY. These conventions include notes, exclusion terms, inclusion terms and definitions for the code designations of Other Specified and Unspecified. There are several additional conventions that appear in the ICF-CY.

1. With reference to the definitions of the negative aspect of Body Functions, Body Structures and Activities/Participation, the term "delay" was added to reflect the fact that a problem in any of these domains may also reflect a lag in development.

2. In a related convention, the concept of delay also denotes the qualifier levels from 0=no delay to 4=complete delay.

4.4 Evidence for coding

The ICF-CY is a classification of Body Functions, Body Structures, Activities and Participation, and Environmental Factors stated in neutral terms. Documentation of a child's problems through the assignment of codes is predicated on the use of the universal qualifier. Assignment of codes must not be based on inference but on explicit information related to the child's functioning problems in the respective domains.

As noted above, evidence for coding can take the form of direct measurement, observation, respondent interview and/or professional judgement. Although the form of the evidence will depend on the characteristic of the function of interest and the purpose for coding, every effort should be made to obtain the most objective information possible. Direct measurement of laboratory, biomedical or anthropometric data constitutes appropriate information for Body Functions and Body Structure. For Activities and Participation, direct measurement may be made with a wide range of standardized instruments and other measures that provide data specific to a domain of interest. In both of these contexts, measurement that is based on normative data can facilitate translation to corresponding qualifier levels in the form of percentile values or standard deviation units. At present, there are instruments and measures that can be used as evidence for assigning codes. However, the correspondence to specific ICF-CY domains is limited. In the search for appropriate instruments, the user is encouraged to select those that have the closest correspondence to these domains of interest and have demonstrated reliability.

Qualitative descriptions of the child, based on direct observation, may be useful in gathering evidence in areas of functioning where assessment instruments are not available or not appropriate. A major goal of the ICF and ICF-CY is to involve respondents in defining the nature and extent of their functioning in the context of their environments. This is especially important when participation is coded. The use of interview is encouraged with children and youth whenever possible. With young children and those with limited verbal skills, the primary caregiver can serve as a proxy respondent. Finally, evidence for coding can be based on professional judgement and on various sources of information including records, observation, and other forms of client contact.

There are several resources that can be drawn upon for evidence in assigning codes. It is beyond the scope of this volume to list instruments and measures for potential use during assessment, but users are encouraged to identify such a list. It may be helpful to review existing measures in reference texts that identify a range of measures applicable to the assessment of Body Functions and Structures, Activities and Participation, and Environmental Factors. Users are encouraged to access reference texts describing instruments accepted in those countries in which they work. The growing interest in the application of the ICF and ICF-CY is contributing to the identification of applicable instruments as well as to the development of new measures consistent with the framework of the ICF-CY. One helpful resource maybe the *Practice Guideline for Psychiatric Evaluation of Adults* (1995) developed by the American Psychological Association for use in service settings. The practice manual is designed for multidisciplinary use and provides comprehensive guidelines regarding the nature of the information needed to assign codes in each of the domains. Finally, training manuals and courses are increasingly likely to be available with the adoption of the ICF-CY in various settings.

5. Case vignettes

The brief information presented in the case vignettes below is designed to illustrate the source of information that can be used when assigning ICF-CY codes to problems manifested by children. In practice, the nature and complexity of information available about a child would clearly be more comprehensive than in these vignettes. However, for the purpose of illustrating the use of the ICF-CY, the user is encouraged to review the cases and identify codes reflecting the problems characterizing each of the children presented. As an initial step, it may be helpful to review the broad questions below and identify any problems noted in the case description. The user can then proceed with the sequence of steps described in the previous section for assigning ICF-CY codes on the basis of information available about a child. The primary focus should be on identifying relevant codes because the vignettes do not provide sufficient information to assign the level of the qualifier.

1. Is the child or adolescent manifesting problems in body functions?

2. Does the child or adolescent have problems of organ, limb or other body structures?

3. Does the child or adolescent have problems executing tasks or actions?

4. Does the child or adolescent have problems engaging in age appropriate life situations?

5. Are there environmental factors that restrict or facilitate the child's or adolescent's functioning?

Case
3-year-old girl

C is a 3-year-old girl who was born following an uneventful pregnancy. She has a history of congenital heart problems, which were corrected in two surgeries early in life. She continues to have frequent upper respiratory and ear infections, which appear to have affected her hearing.

C and her mother live in an apartment in the centre of a large city and receive their medical care from a clinic at one of the city's hospitals. C's father left shortly after her birth and does not contribute to the family financially. C is cared for by a neighbour during the day while her mother works at a local store. When her mother works on the weekends, C stays at her grandmother's with her siblings. C is a serious child who does not smile or laugh easily. She spends much of the time in simple play with objects by herself and does not interact much with other children. She likes things that make noise when they are pushed or pulled and will play with them for long periods of time. Other than that, she is easily distracted. When her attention is not engaged, she is inclined to engage in body rocking. She started walking only three months ago and is unable to climb stairs unless someone is holding her hand. She has a vocabulary of about 20 words that are intelligible, such as "mine", "more", "block", "juice", and a larger vocabulary that is unintelligible. Sitting on her mother's lap to be read a story is one of her favourite activities. She will point to familiar pictures but has difficulty learning the names of objects in the pictures. Frequently, when her name is called, she does not respond and often seems unaware of people talking around her. The basis for these behaviours is unclear but may be due to hearing loss from frequent ear infections. An assessment conducted when she was 24 months old revealed that her developmental level was equivalent to 17 months. Particular delay was evident in receptive and expressive language. Hearing assessment revealed mild, bilateral hearing loss.

With reference to the five questions defined above, the problems manifested by this child suggests codes in Chapters 1, 2, 4 and 7 of the Body Functions component. For Activities and Participation, applicable codes could be considered from Chapters 1, 3, 4, 7 and 8. Codes defining the nature of barriers and facilitators in this child's situation would include some found in Chapters 1 and 3 of the Environmental Factors component.

Case
10-year-old boy

T is a ten-year-old boy who was referred to a clinic for an evaluation after experiencing pervasive academic difficulties in the previous two years of school. On the basis of observation, it is clear that he has significant problems in concentrating on academic tasks and is easily distracted. His parents report that T is "on the go" all the time and does not seem to listen. According to his parents and teachers, he has difficulty keeping still for any length of time at home and at school. At the present time, this means that he has trouble completing assigned work in the classroom. He has particular difficulties remembering material he has studied. He is currently failing all of his academic classes and his performance in reading and writing is at the second grade level. He also shows difficulties adjusting to social situations involving other children.

T's teacher and parents are concerned about his high level of activity and the fact that he does not seem to be able to think before he acts. This is evident in his social behaviour when he fails to wait for his turn in games and sports and, at home, when he rides his bicycle into a busy street without looking. A number of different interventions have been tried to help T perform in the classroom, but these have not resulted in improved performance. While the family has been reluctant to consider medication, T was recently seen by his paediatrician who prescribed a stimulant medication for his high level of activity. In conjunction with the medication trial, the school is designing a comprehensive plan to support T in the classroom.

The problems presented by this 10-year-old boy encompass a number of codes in Chapter 1 of the Body Functions component. For the Activities and Participation component, Chapters 1, 2, 3, 7 and 8 contain codes applicable to document his elevated level of activity and difficulties in meeting the situational and academic demands of the classroom. Applicable codes to describe relevant Environmental Factors would include some found in Chapters 1 and 5.

Case
14-year-old adolescent

J is a 14-year-old girl living with her parents in a small town. She has severe asthma which was detected at a very young age. In addition to heightened response to specific allergens, J's asthmatic attacks are also triggered by exercise, cold air and anxiety. These attacks last 1 to 2 hours and occur several times a week. She is currently prescribed a bronchodilator and uses a nebulizer prophylactically. In the last year, however, J has been inconsistent in following the medication regimen with the result that acute episodes are occurring more frequently. From the time she was enrolled in a preschool programme to the present, J's school attendance has been marked by frequent absences. As a result, her achievement levels have been consistently poor and, while she has not failed any grades, she is falling farther and farther behind her peers.

At the present time, she is in the eighth grade in the local middle school. As exercise triggers acute episodes, she does not participate in the physical education programme at school and does not undertake any regular physical activity. She is frequently absent from school, remaining at home where she watches television and eats snacks. She has gained a significant amount of weight in the last year. Because of frequent absences, J has not developed a consistent group of friends at school. J reports feeling different from others and isolated from her peers. Her parents are becoming very concerned about her physical and emotional health and are consulting a medical doctor.

The chronic health condition of this adolescent is manifested in problems that would be captured primarily in codes found in Chapters 1, 4 and 5 under the Body Functions component. For the Activities and Participation component, most of the applicable codes would be found in Chapters 2, 5, 7, 8 and 9. Finally, for the significant role of the natural environment and asthma medication as well as associated consequences of social isolation, Chapters 1, 2 and 3 of the Environmental Factors component would yield appropriate codes for the documentation of barriers faced by this young person.

6. Acknowledgements

The Members of the Work Group acknowledge with appreciation the support and contributions made by:

Christian Care Foundation for Children with Disabilities in Thailand (CCD), Nonthaburi, Thailand; Collaborating Centres for the WHO Family of International Classifications (WHO-FIC) and affiliated agencies in Australia, Canada, Denmark, Finland, France, Germany, Iceland, Japan, the Netherlands, Norway, the People's Republic of China, Sweden and the USA; EducAid, Rimini, Italy; Instituto Nazionale Neurologico Carlo Besta, Fondazione IRCCS [Italian National Neurological Institute Carlo Besta IRCCS Foundation], Milan, Italy; Gruppo di ricerca, Istituto di Ricovero e Cura a Carattere Scientifico (IRCCS) "Eugenio Medea", Associazione la Nostra Famiglia [Research Group for the Scientific Institute "Eugenio Medea" for Research, Hospitalization and Health Care, Association "La Nostra Famiglia"], Costamasnaga, Italy; Neuropsychiatric Unit, Treviglio Hospital, Treviglio, Italy; Organismo Volontari Cooperazione Internazional (OVCI-La Nostra Famiglia) [Volunteers Organization for International Cooperation], Usratuna, Juba, Sudan; persons associated with government agencies, public and private programmes for children and youth around the world who participated in field trial activities; regional representatives participating in meetings of the WHO Work Group in South Africa, Sweden, Switzerland, Thailand and the USA; The Centre for Epidemiology, Swedish National Board of Health and Welfare, Stockholm, Sweden; The National Center on Birth Defects and Developmental Disabilities of the US Centers for Disease Control and Prevention, Atlanta, GA, USA; University of North Carolina at Chapel Hill, Chapel Hill NC, USA; University of Zurich, Zurich, Switzerland.

Individuals:

Argentina
Christian Plebst

Australia
Sharynne McLeod

Brazil
Heloisa Dinubila

Canada
Diane Caulfield
Patrick Fougeyrollas
Janice Miller

China
Qiu Zhuoying

Denmark
Tora Dahl

Egypt
Mohammed El Banna

Finland
Markku Leskinen

France
Catherine Barral
Jean-Yves Barreyre
Marie Cuenot

Ghana
Kofi Marfo

Iceland
Halla Tulinius

Italy
Daniela Ajovalasit
Francesca Albanesi
Luigi Barruffo
Mariamalia Battaglia
Daniela Beretta
Debora Bonacina
Gabriella Borri
Giovanni Cattoni

Giovanni Cattoni
Elisa Ceppi
Alessio Chiusso
Annalisa Colpo
Maria Antonella Costantino
Guido Corona
Antonella Dimo
Enrico Gruppi
Guido Fusaro
Felicia Licciardi
Bertilla Magagnin
Elena Maria Mauri
Barbara Orlandi
Sabrina Pasqualotti
Alfredo Pisacane
Camilla Pisoni
Gianni de Polo
Monica Pradal
Alberto Raggi
Daria Riva
Lia Rusca
Emanuela Russo
Carlo Sorella
Antonella Vaudano
Anna Zana

Japan
Yutaka Sakai
Akio Tokunaga

Kuwait
Hashem Taqi

Mexico
Fabiola Barron

Peru
Liliana Mayo

Portugal
Joaquim Bairrao
Maria Isabel Felgueiras

South Africa
Erna Alant

Spain
Jaime Ponte

Sudan
Sanson Baba
Marco Sala

Sweden
Margareta Adolfsson
Lars Berg
Kristina Bränd Persson
Lilly Eriksson
Mats Granlund
Nina Ibragimova
Mia Pless
Regina Ylvén

Switzerland
Simon Haskell

Thailand
Wasan Saenwian
Chariya Saenwian
Ko-Chih Tung

The former Yugoslav Republic of Macedonia
Bilijana Ancevska
Anica S. Apceva
Sande S. Bojkovski
Katerina Dimitrova
Vasilka S. Dimovska
Ivan S. Dvojakov
Joanis Gajdazis
Teuta Jakupi
Nikola Jankov
Olga Jotovska
Mirjana P. Kjaeva
Saso S. Kocankovski
Petre S. Krstev
Oliviera Lekovska
Lidja S. Parlic
Snezana D. Pejkovska
Anastasija S. Petrova
Marina S. Pop-Lazarova
Marija Raleva
Fulvia V. Tomatis
Milka S. Vancova
Julija S. Vasileva

United States of America
Stephen Bagnato
Scott Brown
Wendy Coster
Marjorie Greenberg
Heidi Feldman

Anita Scarborugh
Travis Threats

Zambia
Elisa Facelli
Sister Irina
Paolo Marelli

ICF

Introduction

1. Background

This volume contains the *International Classification of Functioning, Disability and Health,* known as ICF.[7] The overall aim of the ICF classification is to provide a unified and standard language and framework for the description of health and health-related states. It defines components of health and some health-related components of well-being (such as education and labour). The domains contained in ICF can, therefore, be seen as *health domains* and *health-related domains.* These domains are described from the perspective of the body, the individual and society in two basic lists: (1) Body Functions and Structures; and (2) Activities and Participation.[8] As a classification, ICF systematically groups different domains[9] for a person in a given health condition (e.g. what a person with a disease or disorder does do or can do). *Functioning* is an umbrella term encompassing all body functions, activities and participation; similarly, *disability* serves as an umbrella term for impairments, activity limitations or participation restrictions. ICF also lists environmental factors that interact with all these constructs. In this way, it enables the user to record useful profiles of individuals' functioning, disability and health in various domains.

ICF belongs to the "family" of international classifications developed by the World Health Organization (WHO) for application to various aspects of health. The WHO family of international classifications provides a framework to code a wide range of information about health (e.g. diagnosis, functioning and disability, reasons for contact with health services) and uses a standardized common language permitting communication about health and health care across the world in various disciplines and sciences.

In WHO's international classifications, health conditions (diseases, disorders, injuries, etc.) are classified primarily in ICD-10 (shorthand for the International Classification of Diseases, Tenth Revision),[10] which provides an etiological framework. Functioning and disability

---

[7] The text represents a revision of the International Classification of Impairments, Disabilities, and Handicaps (ICIDH), which was first published by the World Health Organization for trial purposes in 1980. Developed after systematic field trials and international consultation over the past five years, it was endorsed by the Fifty-fourth World Health Assembly for international use on 22 May 2001 (resolution WHA54.21).

[8] These terms, which replace the formerly used terms "impairment", "disability" and "handicap" , extend the scope of the classification to allow positive experiences to be described. The new terms are further defined in this Introduction and are detailed within the classification. It should be noted that these terms are used with specific meanings that may differ from their everyday usage.

[9] A domain is a pactical and meaningful set of related physiological functions, anatomical structures, actions, tasks, or areas of life.

[10] International Statistical Classification of Diseases and Related Health Problems, Tenth Revision, Vols. 1-3. Geneva, World Health Organization, 1992-1994.

associated with health conditions are classified in ICF. ICD-10 and ICF are therefore complementary,[11] and users are encouraged to utilize these two members of the WHO family of international classifications together. ICD-10 provides a "diagnosis" of diseases, disorders or other health conditions, and this information is enriched by the additional information given by ICF on functioning.[12] Together, information on diagnosis plus functioning provides a broader and more meaningful picture of the health of people or populations, which can then be used for decision-making purposes.

The WHO family of international classifications provides a valuable tool to describe and compare the health of populations in an international context. The information on mortality (provided by ICD-10) and on health outcomes (provided by ICF) may be combined in summary measures of population health for monitoring the health of populations and its distribution, and also for assessing the contributions of different causes of mortality and morbidity.

ICF has moved away from being a "consequences of disease" classification (1980 version) to become a "components of health" classification. "Components of health" identifies the constituents of health, whereas "consequences" focuses on the impacts of diseases or other health conditions that may follow as a result. Thus, ICF takes a neutral stand with regard to etiology so that researchers can draw causal inferences using appropriate scientific methods. Similarly, this approach is also different from a "determinants of health" or "risk factors" approach. To facilitate the study of determinants or risk factors, ICF includes a list of environmental factors that describe the context in which individuals live.

---

[11] It is also important to recognize the overlap between ICD-10 and ICF. Both classifications begin with the body systems. Impairments refer to body structures and functions, which are usually parts of the "disease process" and are therefore also used in the ICD-10. Nevertheless, ICD-10 uses impairments (as signs and symptoms) as parts of a constellation that forms a "disease", or sometimes as reasons for contact with health services, whereas the ICF system uses impairments as problems of body functions and structures associated with health conditions.

[12] Two persons with the same disease can have different levels of functioning, and two persons with the same level of functioning do not necessarily have the same health condition. Hence, joint use enhances data quality for medical purposes. Use of ICF should not bypass regular diagnostic procedures. In other uses, ICF may be used alone.

2. Aims of ICF

ICF is a multipurpose classification designed to serve various disciplines and different sectors. Its specific aims can be summarized as follows:

- to provide a scientific basis for understanding and studying health and health-related states, outcomes and determinants;

- to establish a common language for describing health and health-related states in order to improve communication between different users, such as health-care workers, researchers, policy-makers and the public, including people with disabilities;

- to permit comparison of data across countries, health-care disciplines, services and time;

- to provide a systematic coding scheme for health information systems.

These aims are interrelated, since the need for and uses of ICF require the construction of a meaningful and practical system that can be used by various consumers for health policy, quality assurance and outcome evaluation in different cultures.

2.1 Applications of ICF

Since its publication as a trial version in 1980, ICIDH has been used for various purposes, for example:

- as a statistical tool – in the collection and recording of data (e.g. in population studies and surveys or in management information systems);

- as a research tool – to measure outcomes, quality of life or environmental factors;

- as a clinical tool – in needs assessment, matching treatments with specific conditions, vocational assessment, rehabilitation and outcome evaluation;

- as a social policy tool – in social security planning, compensation systems and policy design and implementation;

- as an educational tool – in curriculum design and to raise awareness and undertake social action.

Since ICF is inherently a health and health-related classification it is also used by sectors such as insurance, social security, labour, education, economics, social policy and general legislation development, and environmental modification. It has been accepted as one of the United Nations social classifications and is referred to in and incorporates *The Standard Rules on the Equalization of Opportunities for Persons with Disabilities*.[13] Thus, ICF provides an appropriate instrument for the implementation of stated international human rights mandates as well as national legislation.

---

[13] *The Standard Rules on the Equalization of Opportunities for Persons with Disabilities*. Adopted by the United Nations General Assembly at its 48th session on 20 December 1993 (resolution 48/96). New York, NY, United Nations Department of Public Information, 1994.

ICF is useful for a broad spectrum of different applications, for example social security, evaluation in managed health care, and population surveys at local, national and international levels. It offers a conceptual framework for information that is applicable to personal health care, including prevention, health promotion, and the improvement of participation by removing or mitigating societal hindrances and encouraging the provision of social supports and facilitators. It is also useful for the study of health-care systems, in terms of both evaluation and policy formulation.

3. Properties of ICF

A classification should be clear about what it classifies: its universe, its scope, its units of classification, its organization, and how these elements are structured in terms of their relation to each other. The following sections explain these basic properties of ICF.

3.1 Universe of ICF

ICF encompasses all aspects of human health and some health-relevant components of well-being and describes them in terms of *health domains* and *health-related domains*.[14] The classification remains in the broad context of health and does not cover circumstances that are not health-related, such as those brought about by socioeconomic factors. For example, because of their race, gender, religion or other socioeconomic characteristics people may be restricted in their execution of a task in their current environment, but these are not health-related restrictions of participation as classified in ICF.

There is a widely held misunderstanding that ICF is only about people with disabilities; in fact, it is about *all people*. The health and health-related states associated with all health conditions can be described using ICF. In other words, ICF has universal application.[15]

3.2 Scope of ICF

ICF provides a description of situations with regard to human functioning and its restrictions and serves as a framework to organize this information. It structures the information in a meaningful, interrelated and easily accessible way.

ICF organizes information in two parts. Part 1 deals with Functioning and Disability, while Part 2 covers Contextual Factors. Each part has two components.

1. Components of Functioning and Disability

The **Body** component comprises two classifications, one for functions of body systems, and one for body structures. The chapters in both classifications are organized according to the body systems.

The **Activities and Participation** component covers the complete range of domains denoting aspects of functioning from both an individual and a societal perspective.

2. Components of Contextual Factors

A list of **Environmental Factors** is the first component of Contextual Factors. Environmental factors have an impact on all components of functioning and disability and are organized in sequence from the individual's most immediate environment to the general environment.

---

[14] Examples of health domains include seeing, hearing, walking, learning and remembering, while examples of health-related domains include transportation, education and social interactions.

[15] Bickenbach JE, Chatterji S, Badley EM, Üstün TB. Models of disablement, universalism and the ICIDH, *Social Science and Medicine*, 1999, 48:1173-1187.

Personal Factors is also a component of Contextual Factors but they are not classified in ICF because of the large social and cultural variance associated with them.

The components of Functioning and Disability in Part 1 of ICF can be expressed in two ways. On the one hand, they can be used to indicate problems (e.g. impairment, activity limitation or participation restriction summarized under the umbrella term *disability*); on the other hand, they can indicate nonproblematic (i.e. neutral) aspects of health and health-related states summarized under the umbrella term *functioning).*

These components of functioning and disability are interpreted by means of four separate but related *constructs.* These constructs are operationalized by using *qualifiers.* Body functions and structures can be interpreted by means of changes in physiological systems or in anatomical structures. For the Activities and Participation component, two constructs are available: *capacity* and *performance* (see section 4.2).

A person's functioning and disability is conceived as a dynamic interaction[16] between health conditions (diseases, disorders, injuries, traumas, etc.) and contextual factors. As indicate above, Contextual Factors include both personal and environmental factors. ICF includes a comprehensive list of environmental factors as an essential component of the classification. Environmental factors interact with all the components of functioning and disability. The basic construct of the Environmental Factors component is the facilitating or hindering impact of features of the physical, social and attitudinal world.

3.3 Unit of classification

ICF classifies health and health-related states. The unit of classification is, therefore, *categories* within health and health-related domains. It is important to note, therefore, that in ICF persons are not the units of classification; that is, ICF does not classify people, but describes the situation of each person within an array of health or health-related domains. Moreover, the description is always made within the context of environmental and personal factors.

3.4 Presentation of ICF

ICF is presented in two versions in order to meet the needs of different users for varying levels of detail.

The *full version* of ICF, as contained in this volume, provides classification at four levels of detail. These four levels can be aggregated into a higher-level classification system that includes all the domains at the second level. The two-level system is also available as a *short version* of ICF.

---

[16] This interaction can be viewed as a *process* or a *result* depending on the user.

4. Overview of ICF components

DEFINITIONS[17]

In the context of health:

Body functions are the physiological functions of body systems (including psychological functions).

Body structures are anatomical parts of the body such as organs, limbs and their components.

Impairments are problems in body function or structure such as a significant deviation or loss.

Activity is the execution of a task or action by an individual.

Participation is involvement in a life situation.

Activity limitations are difficulties an individual may have in executing activities.

Participation restrictions are problems an individual may experience in involvement in life situations.

Environmental factors make up the physical, social and attitudinal environment in which people live and conduct their lives.

An overview of these concepts is given in Table 1; they are explained further in operational terms in section 5.1. As the table indicates:

- ICF has two *parts*, each with two *components:*

    Part 1. Functioning and Disability

        (a)   Body Functions and Structures

        (b)   Activities and Participation

    Part 2. Contextual Factors

        (c)   Environmental Factors

        (d)   Personal Factors.

- Each component can be expressed in both *positive* and *negative* terms.

---

[17] See also Annex 1, Taxonomic and Terminological Issues.

- Each component consists of various domains and, within each domain, categories, which are the units of classification. Health and health-related states of an individual may be recorded by selecting the appropriate category code or codes and then adding *qualifiers*, which are numeric codes that specify the extent or the magnitude of the functioning or disability in that category, or the extent to which an environmental factor is a facilitator or barrier.

Table 1. An overview of ICF

	Part 1: Functioning and Disability		Part 2: Contextual Factors	
Components	Body Functions and Structures	Activities and Participation	Environmental Factors	Personal Factors
Domains	Body functions Body structures	Life areas (tasks, actions)	External influences on functioning and disability	Internal influences on functioning and disability
Constructs	Change in body functions (physiological) Change in body structures (anatomical)	Capacity Executing tasks in a standard environment Performance Executing tasks in the current environment	Facilitating or hindering impact of features of the physical, social, and attitudinal world	Impact of attributes of the person
Positive aspect	Functional and structural integrity	Activities Participation	Facilitators	not applicable
	Functioning			
Negative aspect	Impairment	Activity limitation Participation restriction	Barriers / hindrances	not applicable
	Disability			

4.1 Body Functions and Structures and impairments

Definitions: **Body functions** *are the physiological functions of body systems (including psychological functions).*

> *Body structures* are anatomical parts of the body such as organs, limbs and their components.
>
> *Impairments* are problems in body function or structure as a significant deviation or loss.

(1) Body functions and body structures are classified in two different sections. These two classifications are designed for use in parallel. For example, body functions include basic human senses such as "seeing functions" and their structural correlates exist in the form of "eye and related structures".

(2) "Body" refers to the human organism as a whole; hence, it includes the brain and its functions, i.e. the mind. Mental (or psychological) functions are therefore subsumed under body functions.

(3) Body functions and structures are classified according to body systems; consequently, body structures are not considered as organs.[18]

(4) Impairments of structure can involve an anomaly, defect, loss or other significant deviation in body structures. Impairments have been conceptualized in congruence with biological knowledge at the level of tissues or cells and at the subcellular or molecular level. For practical reasons, however, these levels are not listed.[19] The biological foundations of impairments have guided the classification and there may be room for expanding the classification at the cellular or molecular levels. For medical users, it should be noted that impairments are not the same as the underlying pathology, but are the manifestations of that pathology.

(5) Impairments represent a deviation from certain generally accepted population standards in the biomedical status of the body and its functions, and definition of their constituents is undertaken primarily by those qualified to judge physical and mental functioning according to these standards.

(6) Impairments can be temporary or permanent; progressive, regressive or static; intermittent or continuous. The deviation from the population norm may be slight or severe and may fluctuate over time. These characteristics are captured in further descriptions, mainly in the codes, by means of qualifiers after the point.

(7) Impairments are not contingent on etiology or how they are developed; for example, loss of vision or a limb may arise from a genetic abnormality or an injury. The presence of an impairment necessarily implies a cause; however, the cause may not be sufficient to explain the resulting impairment. Also, when there is an impairment, there is a dysfunction in body functions or structures, but this may be related to any of the various diseases, disorders or physiological states.

---

[18] Although organ level was mentioned in the 1980 version of ICIDH, the definition of an "organ" is not clear. The eye and ear are traditionally considered as organs; however, it is difficult to identify and define their boundaries, and the same is true of extremities and internal organs. Instead of an approach by "organ", which implies the existence of an entity or unit within the body, ICF replaces this term with "body structure".

[19] Thus impairments coded using the full version of ICF should be detectable or noticeable by others or the person concerned by direct observation or by inference from observation.

(8)   Impairments may be part or an expression of a health condition, but do not necessarily indicate that a disease is present or that the individual should be regarded as sick.

(9)   Impairments are broader and more inclusive in scope than disorders or diseases; for example, the loss of a leg is an impairment of body structure, but not a disorder or a disease.

(10) Impairments may result in other impairments; for example, a lack of muscle power may impair movement functions, heart functions may relate to deficit in respiratory functions, and impaired perception may relate to thought functions.

(11) Some categories of the Body Functions and Structures component and the ICD-10 categories seem to overlap, particularly with regard to symptoms and signs. However, the purposes of the two classifications are different. ICD-10 classifies symptoms in special chapters to document morbidity or service utilization, whereas ICF shows them as part of the body functions, which may be used for prevention or identifying patients' needs. Most importantly, in ICF the Body Functions and Structures classification is intended to be used along with the Activities and Participation categories.

(12) Impairments are classified in the appropriate categories using defined identification criteria (e.g. as present or absent according to a threshold level). These criteria are the same for body functions and structures. They are: (a) loss or lack; (b) reduction; (c) addition or excess; and (d) deviation. Once an impairment is present, it may be scaled in terms of its severity using the generic qualifier in the ICF.

(13) Environmental factors interact with body functions, as in the interactions between air quality and breathing, light and seeing, sounds and hearing, distracting stimuli and attention, ground texture and balance, and ambient temperature and body temperature regulation.

4.2   Activities and Participation /activity limitations and participation restrictions

Definitions: **Activity** *is the execution of a task or action by an individual.*

> **Participation** *is involvement in a life situation.*

> **Activity limitations** *are difficulties an individual may have in executing activities.*

> **Participation restrictions** *are problems an individual may experience in involvement in life situations.*

(1)   The domains for the Activities and Participation component are given in a *single list* that covers the full range of life areas (from basic learning or watching to composite areas such as interpersonal interactions or employment). The component can be used to denote activities (a) or participation (p) or both. The domains of this component are qualified by the two qualifiers of *performance* and *capacity*. Hence, the information gathered from the list provides a data matrix that has no overlap or redundancy (see Table 2).

Table 2. Activities and Participation: information matrix

Domains		Qualifiers	
		Performance	Capacity
d1	Learning and applying knowledge		
d2	General tasks and demands		
d3	Communication		
d4	Mobility		
d5	Self-care		
d6	Domestic life		
d7	Interpersonal interactions and relationships		
d8	Major life areas		
d9	Community, social and civic life		

(2) The *performance* qualifier describes what an individual does in his or her current environment. Because the current environment includes a societal context, performance can also be understood as "involvement in a life situation" or "the lived experience" of people in the actual context in which they live.[20] This context includes the environmental factors – all aspects of the physical, social and attitudinal world, which can be coded using the Environmental Factors component.

(3) The *capacity* qualifier describes an individual's ability to execute a task or an action. This construct aims to indicate the highest probable level of functioning that a person may reach in a given domain at a given moment. To assess the full ability of the individual, one would need to have a "standardized" environment to neutralize the varying impact of different environments on the ability of the individual. This standardized environment may be: (a) an actual environment commonly used for capacity assessment in test settings; or (b) in cases where this is not possible, an assumed environment which can be thought to have a uniform impact. This environment can be called a "uniform" or "standard" environment. Thus, capacity reflects the environmentally adjusted ability of the individual. This adjustment has to be the same for all persons in all countries to allow for international comparisons. The features of the uniform or standard environment can be coded using the Environmental Factors

---

[20] The definition of "participation" brings in the concept of involvement. Some proposed definitions of "involvement" incorporate taking part, being included or engaged in an area of life, being accepted, or having access to needed resources. Within the information matrix in Table 2, the only possible indicator of participation is coding through performance. This does not mean that participation is automatically equated with performance. The concept of involvement should also be distinguished from the subjective experience of involvement (the sense of "belonging"). Users who wish to code involvement separately should refer to the coding guidelines in Annex 2.

classification. The gap between capacity and performance reflects the difference between the impacts of current and uniform environments and, thus, provides a useful guide as to what can be done to the environment of the individual to improve performance.

(4) Both capacity and performance qualifiers can also be used with and without assistive devices or personal assistance. While neither devices nor personal assistance eliminate the impairments, they may remove limitations on functioning in specific domains. This type of coding is particularly useful to identify how much the functioning of the individual would be limited without the assistive devices (see coding guidelines in Annex 2).

(5) Difficulties or problems in these domains can arise when there is a qualitative or quantitative alteration in the way in which an individual carries out these domain functions. *Limitations* or *restrictions* are assessed against a generally accepted population standard. The standard or norm against which an individual's capacity and performance is compared is that of an individual without a similar health condition (disease, disorder or injury, etc.). The limitation or restriction records the discordance between the observed and the expected performance. The expected performance is the population norm, which represents the experience of people without the specific health condition. The same norm is used in the capacity qualifier so that one can infer what can be done to the environment of the individual to enhance performance.

(6) A problem with performance can result directly from the social environment, even when the individual has no impairment. For example, an individual who is HIV-positive without any symptoms or disease, or someone with a genetic predisposition to a certain disease, may exhibit no impairments or may have sufficient capacity to work, yet may not do so because of the denial of access to services, discrimination or stigma.

(7) It is difficult to distinguish between "Activities" and "Participation" on the basis of the domains in the Activities and Participation component. Similarly, differentiating between "individual" and "societal" perspectives on the basis of domains has not been possible given international variation and differences in the approaches of professionals and theoretical frameworks. Therefore, ICF provides a single list that can be used, if users so wish, to differentiate activities and participation in their own operational ways. This is further explained in Annex 3. There are four possible ways of doing so:

    (a) to designate some domains as activities and others as participation, not allowing any overlap;

    (b) same as (a) above, but allowing partial overlap;

    (c) to designate all detailed domains as activities and the broad category headings as participation;

    (d) to use all domains as both activities and participation.

4.3 Contextual Factors

Contextual Factors represent the complete background of an individual's life and living. They include two components: Environmental Factors and Personal Factors, which may have an impact on the individual with a health condition and that individual's health and health-related states.

Environmental factors make up the physical, social and attitudinal environment in which people live and conduct their lives. These factors are external to individuals and can have a positive or negative influence on the individual's performance as a member of society, on the individual's capacity to execute actions or tasks, or on the individual's body function or structure.

(1) Environmental factors are organized in the classification to focus on two different levels.

    (a) *Individual* – in the immediate environment of the individual, including settings such as home, workplace and school. Included at this level are the physical and material features of the environment that an individual comes face to face with, as well as direct contact with others such as family, acquaintances, peers and strangers.

    (b) *Societal* – formal and informal social structures, services and overarching approaches or systems in the community or society that have an impact on individuals. This level includes organizations and services related to the work environment, community activities, government agencies, communication and transportation services, and informal social networks as well as laws, regulations, formal and informal rules, attitudes and ideologies.

(2) Environmental factors interact with the components of Body Functions and Structures and Activities and Participation. For each component, the nature and extent of that interaction may be elaborated by future scientific work. Disability is characterized as the outcome or result of a complex relationship between an individual's health condition and personal factors, and of the external factors that represent the circumstances in which the individual lives. Because of this relationship, different environments may have a very different impact on the same individual with a given health condition. An environment with barriers, or without facilitators, will restrict the individual's performance; other environments that are more facilitating may increase that performance. Society may hinder an individual's performance because either it creates barriers (e.g. inaccessible buildings) or it does not provide facilitators (e.g. unavailability of assistive devices).

Personal factors are the particular background of an individual's life and living, and comprise features of the individual that are not part of a health condition or health states. These factors may include gender, race, age, other health conditions, fitness, lifestyle, habits, upbringing, coping styles, social background, education, profession, past and current experience (past life events and concurrent events), overall behaviour pattern and character style, individual psychological assets and other characteristics, all or any of which may play a role in disability at any level. Personal factors are not classified in ICF. However, they are included in Fig. 1 to show their contribution, which may have an impact on the outcome of various interventions.

5. Model of Functioning and Disability

5.1 Process of functioning and disability

As a classification, ICF does not model the "process" of functioning and disability. It can be used, however, to describe the process by providing the means to map the different constructs and domains. It provides a multi-perspective approach to the classification of functioning and disability as an interactive and evolutionary process. It provides the building blocks for users who wish to create models and study different aspects of this process. In this sense, ICF can be seen as a language: the texts that can be created with it depend on the users, their creativity and their scientific orientation. In order to visualize the current understanding of interaction of various components, the diagram presented in Fig. 1 may be helpful.[21]

Fig. 1. Interactions between the components of ICF

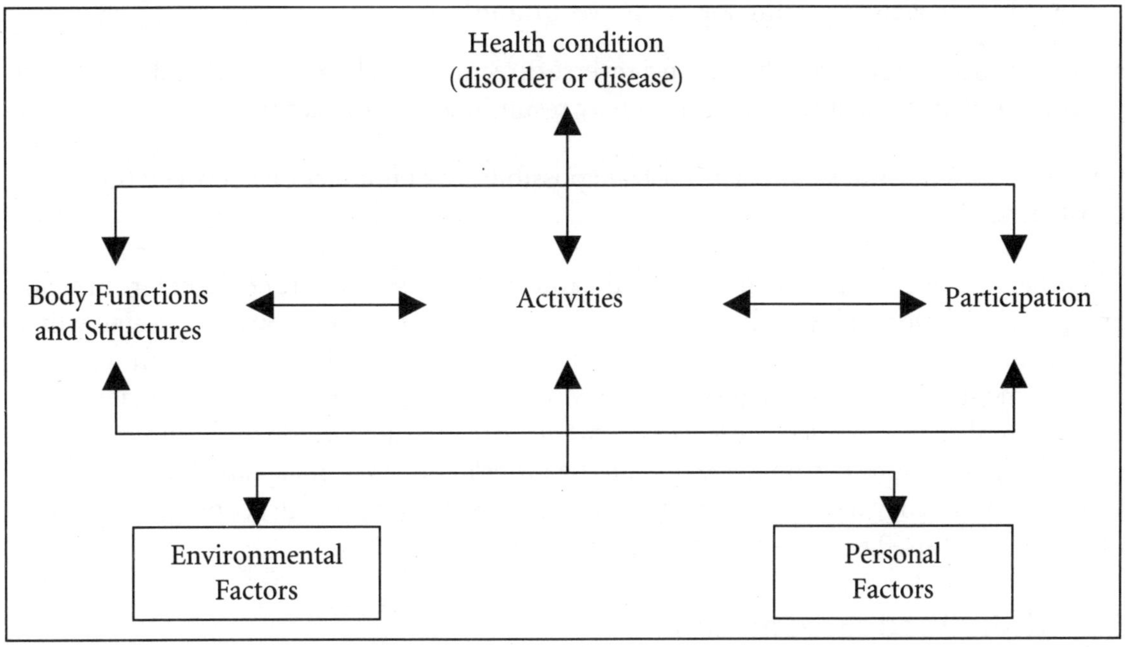

In this diagram, an individual's functioning in a specific domain is an interaction or complex relationship between the health condition and contextual factors (i.e. environmental and personal factors). There is a dynamic interaction among these entities: interventions in one entity have the potential to modify one or more of the other entities. These interactions are specific and not always in a predictable one-to-one relationship. The interaction works in two directions; the presence of disability may even modify the health condition itself. To infer a limitation in capacity from one or more impairments, or a restriction of performance

---

[21] ICF differs substantially from the 1980 version of ICIDH in the depiction of the interrelations between functioning and disability. It should be noted that any diagram is likely to be incomplete and prone to misrepresentation because of the complexity of interactions in a multidimensional model. The model is drawn to illustrate multiple interactions. Other depictions indicating other important foci in the process are certainly possible. Interpretations of interactions between different components and constructs may also vary (for example, the impact of environmental factors on body functions certainly differs from their impact on participation).

from one or more limitations, may often seem reasonable. It is important, however, to collect data on these constructs independently and thereafter explore associations and causal links between them. If the full health experience is to be described, all components are useful. For example, one may:

- have impairments without having capacity limitations (e.g. a disfigurement in leprosy may have no effect on a person's capacity);

- have performance problems and capacity limitations without evident impairments (e.g. reduced performance in daily activities associated with many diseases);

- have performance problems without impairments or capacity limitations (e.g. an HIV-positive individual, or an ex-patient recovered from mental illness, facing stigmatization or discrimination in interpersonal relations or work);

- have capacity limitations without assistance, and no performance problems in the current environment (e.g. an individual with mobility limitations may be provided by society with assistive technology to move around);

- experience a degree of influence in a reverse direction (e.g. lack of use of limbs can cause muscle atrophy; institutionalization may result in loss of social skills).

Case examples in Annex 4 further illustrate possibilities of interactions between the constructs.

The scheme shown in Fig. 1 demonstrates the role that contextual factors (i.e. environmental and personal factors) play in the process. These factors interact with the individual with a health condition and determine the level and extent of the individual's functioning. Environmental factors are extrinsic to the individual (e.g. the attitudes of the society, architectural characteristics, the legal system) and are classified in the Environmental Factors classification. Personal Factors, on the other hand, are not classified in the current version of ICF. They include gender, race, age, fitness, lifestyle, habits, coping styles and other such factors. Their assessment is left to the user, if needed.

5.2 Medical and social models

A variety of conceptual models[22] has been proposed to understand and explain disability and functioning. These may be expressed in a dialectic of "medical model" versus "social model". The *medical model* views disability as a problem of the person, directly caused by disease, trauma or other health condition, which requires medical care provided in the form of individual treatment by professionals. Management of the disability is aimed at cure or the individual's adjustment and behaviour change. Medical care is viewed as the main issue, and at the political level the principal response is that of modifying or reforming health care policy. The *social model* of disability, on the other hand, sees the issue mainly as a socially created problem, and basically as a matter of the full integration of individuals into society. Disability is not an attribute of an individual, but rather a complex collection of conditions, many of which are created by the social environment. Hence, the management of the problem requires social action, and it is the collective responsibility of society at large to

---

[22] The term "model" here means construct or paradigm, which differs from the use of the term in the previous section.

make the environmental modifications necessary for the full participation of people with disabilities in all areas of social life. The issue is, therefore, an attitudinal or ideological one requiring social change, which at the political level becomes a question of human rights. For this model disability is a political issue.

ICF is based on an integration of these two opposing models. In order to capture the integration of the various perspectives of functioning, a "biopsychosocial" approach is used. Thus, ICF attempts to achieve a synthesis, in order to provide a coherent view of different perspectives of health from a biological, individual and social perspective.[23]

---

[23] See also Annex 5 – "ICF and people with disabilities".

6. Use of ICF

ICF is a classification of human functioning and disability. It systematically groups health and health-related domains. Within each component, domains are further grouped according to their common characteristics (such as their origin, type, or similarity) and ordered in a meaningful way. The classification is organized according to a set of principles (see Annex 1). These principles refer to the interrelatedness of the levels and the hierarchy of the classification (sets of levels). However, some categories in ICF are arranged in a non-hierarchical manner, with no ordering but as equal members of a branch.

The following are structural features of the classification that have a bearing on its use.

(1) ICF gives standard operational definitions of the health and health-related domains as opposed to "vernacular" definitions of health. These definitions describe the essential attributes of each domain (e.g. qualities, properties and relationships) and contain information as to what is included and excluded in each domain. The definitions contain commonly used anchor points for assessment so that they can be translated into questionnaires. Conversely, results from existing assessment instruments can be coded in ICF terms. For example, "seeing functions" are defined in terms of functions of sensing form and contour, from varying distances, using one or both eyes, so that the severity of difficulties of vision can be coded at mild, moderate, severe or total levels in relation to these parameters.

(2) ICF uses an alphanumeric system in which the letters b, s, d and e are used to denote Body Functions, Body Structures, Activities and Participation, and Environmental Factors. These letters are followed by a numeric code that starts with the chapter number (one digit), followed by the second level (two digits), and the third and fourth levels (one digit each).

(3) ICF categories are "nested" so that broader categories are defined to include more detailed subcategories of the parent category. For example, Chapter 4 on Mobility in the Activities and Participation component includes separate categories on standing, sitting, walking, carrying items, and so on. The short (concise) version covers two levels, whereas the full (detailed) version extends to four levels. The short version and full version codes are in correspondence, and the short version can be aggregated from the full version.

(4) Any individual may have a range of codes at each level. These may be independent or interrelated.

(5) The ICF codes are only complete with the presence of a *qualifier*, which denotes a magnitude of the level of health (e.g. severity of the problem). Qualifiers are coded as one, two or more numbers after a point (or *separator*). Use of any code should be accompanied by at least one qualifier. Without qualifiers, codes have no inherent meaning.

(6) The first qualifier for Body Functions and Structures, the performance and capacity qualifiers for Activities and Participation, and the first qualifier for Environmental Factors all describe the extent of problems in the respective component.

(7) All three components classified in ICF (Body Functions and Structures, Activities and Participation, and Environmental Factors) are quantified using the same generic scale.

Having a problem may mean an impairment, limitation, restriction or barrier depending on the construct. Appropriate qualifying words as shown in brackets below should be chosen according to the relevant classification domain (where xxx stands for the second-level domain number). For this quantification to be used in a universal manner, assessment procedures need to be developed through research. Broad ranges of percentages are provided for those cases in which calibrated assessment instruments or other standards are available to quantify the impairment, capacity limitation, performance problem or barrier. For example, when "no problem" or "complete problem" is specified the coding has a margin of error of up to 5%. "Moderate problem" is defined as up to half of the time or half the scale of total difficulty. The percentages are to be calibrated in different domains with reference to relevant population standards as percentiles.

xxx.0 NO problem	(none, absent, negligible,…)	0-4 %
xxx.1 MILD problem	(slight, low,…)	5-24 %
xxx.2 MODERATE problem	(medium, fair,…)	25-49 %
xxx.3 SEVERE problem	(high, extreme,…)	50-95 %
xxx.4 COMPLETE problem	(total,…)	96-100 %
xxx.8 not specified		
xxx.9 not applicable		

(8) In the case of environmental factors, this first qualifier can be used to denote either the extent of positive effects of the environment, i.e. facilitators, or the extent of negative effects, i.e. barriers. Both use the same 0-4 scale, but, to denote facilitators, the point is replaced by a plus sign: for example e110+2. Environmental Factors can be coded (a) in relation to each construct individually, or (b) overall, without reference to any individual construct. The first option is preferable, since it identifies the impact and attribution more clearly.

(9) For different users, it might be appropriate and helpful to add other kinds of information to the coding of each item. There are a variety of additional qualifiers that could be useful. Table 3 sets out the details of the qualifiers for each component as well as suggested additional qualifiers to be developed.

(10) The descriptions of health and health-related domains refer to their use at a given moment (i.e. as a snapshot). However, use at multiple time points is possible to describe a trajectory over time and process.

(11) In ICF, a person's health and health-related states are given an array of codes that encompass the two parts of the classification. Thus, the maximum number of codes per person can be 34 at the one-digit level (8 body functions, 8 body structures, 9 performance and 9 capacity codes). Similarly, for the two-level items the total number of codes is 362. At more detailed levels, these codes number up to 1424 items. In real-life applications of ICF, a set of 3 to 18 codes may be adequate to describe a case with two-level (three-digit) precision. Generally, the more detailed four-level version is used for specialist services (e.g. rehabilitation outcomes, geriatrics), whereas the two-level classification can be used for surveys and clinical outcome evaluation.

Further coding guidelines are presented in Annex 2. Users are strongly recommended to obtain training in the use of the classification through WHO and its network of collaborating centres.

Table 3. Qualifiers

Components	First qualifier	Second qualifier
Body Functions (b)	Generic qualifier with the negative scale used to indicate the extent or magnitude of an impairment Example: b167.3 to indicate a severe impairment in specific mental functions of language	None
Body Structures (s)	Generic qualifier with the negative scale used to indicate the extent or magnitude of an impairment Example: s730.3 to indicate a severe impairment of the upper extremity	Used to indicate the nature of the change in the respective body structure: 0 no change in structure 1 total absence 2 partial absence 3 additional part 4 aberrant dimensions 5 discontinuity 6 deviating position 7 qualitative changes in structure, including accumulation of fluid 8 not specified 9 not applicable Example: s730.32 to indicate the partial absence of the upper extremity
Activities and Participation (d)	Performance Generic qualifier Problem in the person's current environment Example: d5101.1_ to indicate mild difficulty with bathing the whole body with the use of assistive devices that are available to the person in his or her current environment	Capacity Generic qualifier Limitation without assistance Example: d5101._2 to indicate moderate difficulty with bathing the whole body; implies that there is moderate difficulty without the use of assistive devices or personal help
Environmental Factors (e)	Generic qualifier, with negative and positive scale, to denote extent of barriers and facilitators respectively Example: e130.2 to indicate that products for education are a moderate barrier. Conversely, e130 +2 would indicate that products for education are a moderate facilitator	None

54th World Health Assembly endorsement of ICF for international use

The resolution WHA54.21 reads as follows:

The Fifty-fourth World Health Assembly,

1. ENDORSES the second edition of the International Classification of Impairments, Disabilities and Handicaps (ICIDH), with the title International Classification of Functioning, Disability and Health, henceforth referred to in short as ICF;

2. URGES Member States to use ICF in their research, surveillance and reporting as appropriate, taking into account specific situations in Member States and, in particular, in view of possible future revisions;

3. REQUESTS the Director-General to provide support to Member States, at their request, in making use of ICF.

ICF-CY

One-level classification

List of chapter headings
in the classification

Body functions

Chapter 1	Mental functions
Chapter 2	Sensory functions and pain
Chapter 3	Voice and speech functions
Chapter 4	Functions of the cardiovascular, haematological, immunological and respiratory systems
Chapter 5	Functions of the digestive, metabolic and endocrine systems
Chapter 6	Genitourinary and reproductive functions
Chapter 7	Neuromusculoskeletal and movement-related functions
Chapter 8	Functions of the skin and related structures

Body structures

Chapter 1	Structures of the nervous system
Chapter 2	The eye, ear and related structures
Chapter 3	Structures involved in voice and speech
Chapter 4	Structures of the cardiovascular, immunological and respiratory systems
Chapter 5	Structures related to the digestive, metabolic and endocrine systems
Chapter 6	Structures related to the genitourinary and reproductive systems
Chapter 7	Structures related to movement
Chapter 8	Skin and related structures

Activities and participation

Chapter 1	Learning and applying knowledge
Chapter 2	General tasks and demands
Chapter 3	Communication
Chapter 4	Mobility
Chapter 5	Self-care

Chapter 6   Domestic life

Chapter 7   Interpersonal interactions and relationships

Chapter 8   Major life areas

Chapter 9   Community, social and civic life

Environmental factors

Chapter 1   Products and technology

Chapter 2   Natural environment and human-made changes to environment

Chapter 3   Support and relationships

Chapter 4   Attitudes

Chapter 5   Services, systems and policies

ICF-CY

Two-level classification

List of chapter headings and first branching level
in the classification

BODY FUNCTIONS

Chapter 1 Mental functions

Global mental functions (b110-b139)
b110   Consciousness functions
b114   Orientation functions
b117   Intellectual functions
b122   Global psychosocial functions
b125   Dispositions and intra-personal funtions
b126   Temperament and personality functions
b130   Energy and drive functions
b134   Sleep functions
b139   Global mental functions, other specified and unspecified

Specific mental functions (b140-b189)
b140   Attention functions
b144   Memory functions
b147   Psychomotor functions
b152   Emotional functions
b156   Perceptual functions
b160   Thought functions
b163   Basic cognitive functions
b164   Higher-level cognitive functions
b167   Mental functions of language
b172   Calculation functions
b176   Mental function of sequencing complex movements
b180   Experience of self and time functions
b189   Specific mental functions, other specified and unspecified
b198   Mental functions, other specified
b199   Mental functions, unspecified

Chapter 2 Sensory functions and pain

Seeing and related functions (b210-b229)
b210   Seeing functions
b215   Functions of structures adjoining the eye
b220   Sensations associated with the eye and adjoining structures
b229   Seeing and related functions, other specified and unspecified

Hearing and vestibular functions (b230-b249)
b230   Hearing functions
b235   Vestibular functions
b240   Sensations associated with hearing and vestibular function
b249   Hearing and vestibular functions, other specified and unspecified

Additional sensory functions (b250-b279)
b250   Taste function
b255   Smell function

b260	Proprioceptive function
b265	Touch function
b270	Sensory functions related to temperature and other stimuli
b279	Additional sensory functions, other specified and unspecified

Pain (b280-b289)

b280	Sensation of pain
b289	Sensation of pain, other specified and unspecified
b298	Sensory functions and pain, other specified
b299	Sensory functions and pain, unspecified

Chapter 3 Voice and speech functions

b310	Voice functions
b320	Articulation functions
b330	Fluency and rhythm of speech functions
b340	Alternative vocalization functions
b398	Voice and speech functions, other specified
b399	Voice and speech functions, unspecified

Chapter 4 Functions of the cardiovascular, haematological, immunological and respiratory systems

Functions of the cardiovascular system (b410-b429)

b410	Heart functions
b415	Blood vessel functions
b420	Blood pressure functions
b429	Functions of the cardiovascular system, other specified and unspecified

Functions of the haematological and immunological systems (b430-b439)

b430	Haematological system functions
b435	Immunological system functions
b439	Functions of the haematological and immunological systems, other specified and unspecified

Functions of the respiratory system (b440-b449)

b440	Respiration functions
b445	Respiratory muscle functions
b449	Functions of the respiratory system, other specified and unspecified

Additional functions and sensations of the cardiovascular and respiratory systems (b450-b469)

b450	Additional respiratory functions
b455	Exercise tolerance functions
b460	Sensations associated with cardiovascular and respiratory functions
b469	Additional functions and sensations of the cardiovascular and respiratory systems, other specified and unspecified
b498	Functions of the cardiovascular, haematological, immunological and respiratory systems, other specified

b499   Functions of the cardiovascular, haematological, immunological and respiratory systems, unspecified

Chapter 5 Functions of the digestive, metabolic and endocrine systems

Functions related to the digestive system (b510-b539)
b510   Ingestion functions
b515   Digestive functions
b520   Assimilation functions
b525   Defecation functions
b530   Weight maintenance functions
b535   Sensations associated with the digestive system
b539   Functions related to the digestive system, other specified and unspecified

Functions related to metabolism and the endocrine system (b540-b569)
b540   General metabolic functions
b545   Water, mineral and electrolyte balance functions
b550   Thermoregulatory functions
b555   Endocrine gland functions
b560   Growth maintenance functions
b569   Functions related to metabolism and the endocrine system, other specified and unspecified
b598   Functions of the digestive, metabolic and endocrine systems, other specified
b599   Functions of the digestive, metabolic and endocrine systems, unspecified

Chapter 6 Genitourinary and reproductive functions

Urinary functions (b610-b639)
b610   Urinary excretory functions
b620   Urination functions
b630   Sensations associated with urinary functions
b639   Urinary functions, other specified and unspecified

Genital and reproductive functions (b640-b679)
b640   Sexual functions
b650   Menstruation functions
b660   Procreation functions
b670   Sensations associated with genital and reproductive functions
b679   Genital and reproductive functions, other specified and unspecified
b698   Genitourinary and reproductive functions, other specified
b699   Genitourinary and reproductive functions, unspecified

Chapter 7 Neuromusculoskeletal and movement-related functions

Functions of the joints and bones (b710-b729)
b710   Mobility of joint functions
b715   Stability of joint functions
b720   Mobility of bone functions
b729   Functions of the joints and bones, other specified and unspecified

Muscle functions (b730-b749)

b730   Muscle power functions
b735   Muscle tone functions
b740   Muscle endurance functions
b749   Muscle functions, other specified and unspecified

Movement functions (b750-b789)

b750   Motor reflex functions
b755   Involuntary movement reaction functions
b760   Control of voluntary movement functions
b765   Involuntary movement functions
b770   Gait pattern functions
b780   Sensations related to muscles and movement functions
b789   Movement functions, other specified and unspecified
b798   Neuromusculoskeletal and movement-related functions, other specified
b799   Neuromusculoskeletal and movement-related functions, unspecified

Chapter 8 Functions of the skin and related structures

Functions of the skin (b810-b849)

b810   Protective functions of the skin
b820   Repair functions of the skin
b830   Other functions of the skin
b840   Sensation related to the skin
b849   Functions of the skin, other specified and unspecified

Functions of the hair and nails (b850-b869)

b850   Functions of hair
b860   Functions of nails
b869   Functions of the hair and nails, other specified and unspecified
b898   Functions of the skin and related structures, other specified
b899   Functions of the skin and related structures, unspecified

BODY STRUCTURES

Chapter 1 Structures of the nervous system

s110   Structure of brain
s120   Spinal cord and related structures
s130   Structure of meninges
s140   Structure of sympathetic nervous system
s150   Structure of parasympathetic nervous system
s198   Structure of the nervous system, other specified
s199   Structure of the nervous system, unspecified

Chapter 2 The eye, ear and related structures

s210   Structure of eye socket
s220   Structure of eyeball
s230   Structures around eye
s240   Structure of external ear
s250   Structure of middle ear
s260   Structure of inner ear
s298   Eye, ear and related structures, other specified
s299   Eye, ear and related structures, unspecified

Chapter 3 Structures involved in voice and speech

s310   Structure of nose
s320   Structure of mouth
s330   Structure of pharynx
s340   Structure of larynx
s398   Structures involved in voice and speech, other specified
s399   Structures involved in voice and speech, unspecified

Chapter 4 Structures of the cardiovascular, immunological and respiratory systems

s410   Structure of cardiovascular system
s420   Structure of immune system
s430   Structure of respiratory system
s498   Structures of the cardiovascular, immunological and respiratory systems, other specified
s499   Structures of the cardiovascular, immunological and respiratory systems, unspecified

Chapter 5 Structures related to the digestive, metabolic and endocrine systems

s510   Structure of salivary glands
s520   Structure of oesophagus
s530   Structure of stomach
s540   Structure of intestine
s550   Structure of pancreas

s560   Structure of liver
s570   Structure of gall bladder and ducts
s580   Structure of endocrine glands
s598   Structures related to the digestive, metabolic and endocrine systems, other
         specified
s599   Structures related to the digestive, metabolic and endocrine systems,
         unspecified

Chapter 6 Structures related to the genitourinary and reproductive systems

s610   Structure of urinary system
s620   Structure of pelvic floor
s630   Structure of reproductive system
s698   Structures related to the genitourinary and reproductive systems, other
         specified
s699   Structures related to the genitourinary and reproductive systems, unspecified

Chapter 7 Structures related to movement

s710   Structure of head and neck region
s720   Structure of shoulder region
s730   Structure of upper extremity
s740   Structure of pelvic region
s750   Structure of lower extremity
s760   Structure of trunk
s770   Additional musculoskeletal structures related to movement
s798   Structures related to movement, other specified
s799   Structures related to movement, unspecified

Chapter 8 Skin and related structures

s810   Structure of areas of skin
s820   Structure of skin glands
s830   Structure of nails
s840   Structure of hair
s898   Skin and related structures, other specified
s899   Skin and related structures, unspecifed

ACTIVITIES AND PARTICIPATION

Chapter 1 Learning and applying knowledge

Purposeful sensory experiences (d110-d129)
d110   Watching
d115   Listening
d120   Other purposeful sensing
d129   Purposeful sensory experiences, other specified and unspecified

Basic learning (d130-d159)
d130   Copying
d131   Learning through actions with objects
d132   Acquiring information
d133   Acquiring language
d134   Acquiring additional language
d135   Rehearsing
d137   Acquiring concepts
d140   Learning to read
d145   Learning to write
d150   Learning to calculate
d155   Acquiring skills
d159   Basic learning, other specified and unspecified

Applying knowledge (d160-d179)
d160   Focusing attention
d161   Directing attention
d163   Thinking
d166   Reading
d170   Writing
d172   Calculating
d175   Solving problems
d177   Making decisions
d179   Applying knowledge, other specified and unspecified
d198   Learning and applying knowledge, other specified
d199   Learning and applying knowledge, unspecified

Chapter 2 General tasks and demands

d210   Undertaking a single task
d220   Undertaking multiple tasks
d230   Carrying out daily routine
d240   Handling stress and other psychological demands
d250   Managing one's own behaviour
d298   General tasks and demands, other specified
d299   General tasks and demands, unspecified

Chapter 3 Communication

Communicating - receiving (d310-d329)
d310 Communicating with - receiving - spoken messages
d315 Communicating with - receiving - nonverbal messages
d320 Communicating with - receiving - formal sign language messages
d325 Communicating with - receiving - written messages
d329 Communicating - receiving, other specified and unspecified

Communicating - producing (d330-d349)
d330 Speaking
d331 Pre-talking
d332 Singing
d335 Producing nonverbal messages
d340 Producing messages in formal sign language
d345 Writing messages
d349 Communication - producing, other specified and unspecified

Conversation and use of communication devices and techniques (d350-d369)
d350 Conversation
d355 Discussion
d360 Using communication devices and techniques
d369 Conversation and use of communication devices and techniques, other specified and unspecified
d398 Communication, other specified
d399 Communication, unspecified

Chapter 4 Mobility

Changing and maintaining body position (d410-d429)
d410 Changing basic body position
d415 Maintaining a body position
d420 Transferring oneself
d429 Changing and maintaining body position, other specified and unspecified

Carrying, moving and handling objects (d430-d449)
d430 Lifting and carrying objects
d435 Moving objects with lower extremities
d440 Fine hand use
d445 Hand and arm use
d446 Fine foot use
d449 Carrying, moving and handling objects, other specified and unspecified

Walking and moving (d450-d469)
d450 Walking
d455 Moving around
d460 Moving around in different locations
d465 Moving around using equipment
d469 Walking and moving, other specified and unspecified

Moving around using transportation (d470-d489)

d470   Using transportation
d475   Driving
d480   Riding animals for transportation
d489   Moving around using transportation, other specified and unspecified
d498   Mobility, other specified
d499   Mobility, unspecified

Chapter 5 Self-care

d510   Washing oneself
d520   Caring for body parts
d530   Toileting
d540   Dressing
d550   Eating
d560   Drinking
d570   Looking after one's health
d571   Looking after one's safety
d598   Self-care, other specified
d599   Self-care, unspecified

Chapter 6 Domestic life

Acquisition of necessities (d610-d629)

d610   Acquiring a place to live
d620   Acquisition of goods and services
d629   Acquisition of necessities, other specified and unspecified

Household tasks (d630-d649)

d630   Preparing meals
d640   Doing housework
d649   Household tasks, other specified and unspecified

Caring for household objects and assisting others (d650-d669)

d650   Caring for household objects
d660   Assisting others
d669   Caring for household objects and assisting others, other specified and unspecified
d698   Domestic life, other specified
d699   Domestic life, unspecified

Chapter 7 Interpersonal interactions and relationships

General interpersonal interactions (d710-d729)

d710   Basic interpersonal interactions
d720   Complex interpersonal interactions
d729   General interpersonal interactions, other specified and unspecified

Particular interpersonal relationships (d730-d779)

d730   Relating with strangers
d740   Formal relationships
d750   Informal social relationships
d760   Family relationships
d770   Intimate relationships
d779   Particular interpersonal relationships, other specified and unspecified
d798   Interpersonal interactions and relationships, other specified
d799   Interpersonal interactions and relationships, unspecified

Chapter 8 Major life areas

Education (d810-d839)

d810   Informal education
d815   Preschool education
d816   Preschool life and related activities
d820   School education
d825   Vocational training
d830   Higher education
d835   School life and related activities
d839   Education, other specified and unspecified

Work and employment (d840-d859)

d840   Apprenticeship (work preparation)
d845   Acquiring, keeping and terminating a job
d850   Remunerative employment
d855   Non-remunerative employment
d859   Work and employment, other specified and unspecified

Economic life (d860-d879)

d860   Basic economic transactions
d865   Complex economic transactions
d870   Economic self-sufficiency
d879   Economic life, other specified and unspecified
d880   Engagement in play
d898   Major life areas, other specified
d899   Major life areas, unspecified

Chapter 9 Community, social and civic life

d910   Community life
d920   Recreation and leisure
d930   Religion and spirituality
d940   Human rights
d950   Political life and citizenship
d998   Community, social and civic life, other specified
d999   Community, social and civic life, unspecified

ENVIRONMENTAL FACTORS

Chapter 1 Products and technology

e110	Products or substances for personal consumption
e115	Products and technology for personal use in daily living
e120	Products and technology for personal indoor and outdoor mobility and transportation
e125	Products and technology for communication
e130	Products and technology for education
e135	Products and technology for employment
e140	Products and technology for culture, recreation and sport
e145	Products and technology for the practice of religion and spirituality
e150	Design, construction and building products and technology of buildings for public use
e155	Design, construction and building products and technology of buildings for private use
e160	Products and technology of land development
e165	Assets
e198	Products and technology, other specified
e199	Products and technology, unspecified

Chapter 2 Natural environment and human-made changes to environment

e210	Physical geography
e215	Population
e220	Flora and fauna
e225	Climate
e230	Natural events
e235	Human-caused events
e240	Light
e245	Time-related changes
e250	Sound
e255	Vibration
e260	Air quality
e298	Natural environment and human-made changes to environment, other specified
e299	Natural environment and human-made changes to environment, unspecified

Chapter 3 Support and relationships

e310	Immediate family
e315	Extended family
e320	Friends
e325	Acquaintances, peers colleagues, neighbours and community members
e330	People in positions of authority
e335	People in subordinate positions
e340	Personal care providers and personal assistants
e345	Strangers

e350	Domesticated animals
e355	Health professionals
e360	Other professionals
e398	Support and relationships, other specified
e399	Support and relationships, unspecified

Chapter 4 Attitudes

e410	Individual attitudes of immediate family members
e415	Individual attitudes of extended family members
e420	Individual attitudes of friends
e425	Individual attitudes of acquaintances, peers colleagues, neighbours and community members
e430	Individual attitudes of people in positions of authority
e435	Individual attitudes of people in subordinate positions
e440	Individual attitudes of personal care providers and personal assistants
e445	Individual attitudes of strangers
e450	Individual attitudes of health professionals
e455	Individual attitudes of other professionals
e460	Societal attitudes
e465	Social norms, practices and ideologies
e498	Attitudes, other specified
e499	Attitudes, unspecified

Chapter 5 Services, systems and policies

e510	Services, systems and policies for the production of consumer goods
e515	Architecture and construction services, systems and policies
e520	Open space planning services, systems and policies
e525	Housing services, systems and policies
e530	Utilities services, systems and policies
e535	Communication services, systems and policies
e540	Transportation services, systems and policies
e545	Civil protection services, systems and policies
e550	Legal services, systems and policies
e555	Associations and organizational services, systems and policies
e560	Media services, systems and policies
e565	Economic services, systems and policies
e570	Social security services, systems and policies
e575	General social support services, systems and policies
e580	Health services, systems and policies
e585	Education and training services, systems and policies
e590	Labour and employment services, systems and policies
e595	Political services, systems and policies
e598	Services, systems and policies, other specified
e599	Services, systems and policies, unspecified

ICF-CY

Detailed classification with definitions

All categories within the classification with their definitions,
inclusions and exclusions

BODY FUNCTIONS

Definitions: **Body functions** *are the physiological functions of body systems (including psychological functions).*

> **Impairments** *are problems in body function or structure as a significant deviation or loss.*

During childhood and adolescence, impairments may also take the form of delays or lags in the emergence of body functions during development.

Qualifier

Generic qualifier with the negative scale, used to indicate the extent or magnitude of an impairment:

xxx.0	NO impairment	(none, absent, negligible,...)	0-4 %
xxx.1	MILD impairment	(slight, low,...)	5-24 %
xxx.2	MODERATE impairment	(medium, fair,...)	25-49 %
xxx.3	SEVERE impairment	(high, extreme,...)	50-95 %
xxx.4	COMPLETE impairment	(total,...)	96-100 %
xxx.8	not specified		
xxx.9	not applicable		

Broad ranges of percentages are provided for those cases in which calibrated assessment instruments or other standards are available to quantify the impairment in body function. For example, when "no impairment" or "complete impairment" in body function is coded, this scaling may have margin of error of up to 5%. "Moderate impairment" is generally up to half of the scale of total impairment. The percentages are to be calibrated in different domains with reference to population standards as percentiles. For this quantification to be used in a uniform manner, assessment procedures need to be developed through research.

For a further explanation of coding conventions in ICF, refer to Annex 2.

Chapter 1

Mental functions

This chapter is about the functions of the brain: both global mental functions, such as consciousness, energy and drive, and specific mental functions, such as memory, language and calculation mental functions.

Global mental functions (b110-b139)

b110 Consciousness functions
General mental functions of the state of awareness and alertness, including the clarity and continuity of the wakeful state.

Inclusions: functions of the state, continuity and quality of consciousness; loss of consciousness, coma, vegetative states, fugues, trance states, possession states, pharmacologically-(drug)induced altered consciousness, delirium, stupor

Exclusions: orientation functions (b114); energy and drive functions (b130); sleep functions (b134)

b 1100   State of consciousness
Mental functions that when altered produce states, such as clouding of consciousness, stupor or coma.

b 1101   Continuity of consciousness
Mental functions that produce sustained wakefulness, alertness and awareness and, when disrupted, may produce fugue, trance or other similar states.

b 1102   Quality of consciousness
Mental functions that when altered effect changes in the character of wakeful, alert and aware sentience, such as drug-induced altered states or delirium.

b 1103   Regulation of states of wakefulness
Mental functions regulating the organization of stable states of wakefulness and awareness.

b 1108   Consciousness functions, other specified

b 1109   Consciousness functions, unspecified

b114   **Orientation functions**
General mental functions of knowing and ascertaining one's relation to object, to self, to others, to time and to one's surroundings and space.

Inclusions: functions of orientation to time, space, place and person; orientation to self and others; disorientation to time, place and person

Exclusions: consciousness functions (b110); attention functions (b140); memory functions (b144)

b 1140   **Orientation to time**
Mental functions that produce awareness of today, tomorrow, yesterday, date, month and year.

b 1141   **Orientation to place**
Mental functions that produce awareness of one's location, such as one's immediate surroundings, one's town or country.

b 1142   **Orientation to person**
Mental functions that produce awareness of one's own identity and of individuals in the immediate environment.

b 11420   **Orientation to self**
Mental functions that produce awareness of one's own identity.

b 11421   **Orientation to others**
Mental functions that produce awareness of the identity of other individuals in one's immediate environment.

b 11428   **Orientation to person, other specified**

b 11429   **Orientation to person, unspecified**

b 1143   **Orientation to objects**
Mental functions that produce awareness of objects or features of objects.

b 1144   **Orientation to space**
Mental functions that produce awareness of one's body in relationship to the immediate physical space.

b 1148   **Orientation functions, other specified**

b 1149   **Orientation functions, unspecified**

b117 **Intellectual functions**
General mental functions, required to understand and constructively integrate the various mental functions, including all cognitive functions and their development over the life span.

Inclusions: functions of intellectual growth; intellectual retardation, mental retardation, dementia

Exclusions: memory functions (b144); thought functions (b160); basic cognitive functions (b163); higher-level cognitive functions (b164)

b122 **Global psychosocial functions**
General mental functions, as they develop over the life span, required to understand and constructively integrate the mental functions that lead to the formation of the personal and interpersonal skills needed to establish reciprocal social interactions, in terms of both meaning and purpose.

Inclusion: any difficulty in self-other relationships including attachment

b125 **Dispositions and intra-personal functions**
Disposition to act or react in a particular way, characterizing the personal, behavioural style of an individual that is distinct from others. These behavioural and responses styles are developmental in nature and may be foundational for later patterns of temperament and personality functions.

Remark: The codes on Dispositions and Intra-personal functions can be related to the codes on expression of Temperament and Personality functions (b126). Users may use either or both. The taxonomic properties of these codes and their relationship need to be developed through research.

Inclusion: functions of adaptability, responsivity, activity level, predictability, persistence and approachability

Exclusions: intellectual functions (b117); energy and drive functions (b130); psychomotor functions (b147); emotional functions (b152)

b1250 **Adaptability**
Disposition to act or react to new objects or experiences in an accepting manner rather than a resistant manner.

b1251 **Responsivity**
Disposition to react in a positive rather than negative manner to actual or perceived demand.

b1252 **Activity level**
Disposition to act or react with energy and action rather than lethargy and inaction.

b 1253   Predictability
Disposition to act or react in a predictable and stable manner rather than an erratic or unpredictable manner.

b 1254   Persistence
Disposition to act with an appropriately sustained rather than limited effort.

b 1255   Approachability
Disposition to act in an initiating manner, moving towards persons or things rather than retreating or withdrawing.

b 1258   Dispositions and intra-personal functions, other specified

b 1259   Dispositions and intra-personal functions, unspecified

b 126   Temperament and personality functions
General mental functions of constitutional disposition of the individual to react in a particular way to situations, including the set of mental characteristics that makes the individual distinct from others.

Remark: The codes on Temperament and Personality functions can be related to the codes on expression of Dispositions and Intra-personal functions (b125). Users may use either or both. The taxonomic properties of these codes and their relationship need to be developed through research.

Inclusions: functions of extraversion, introversion, agreeableness, conscientiousness, psychic and emotional stability, and openness to experience; optimism; novelty seeking; confidence; trustworthiness

Exclusions: intellectual functions (b117); energy and drive functions (b130); psychomotor functions (b147); emotional functions (b152)

b 1260   Extraversion
Mental functions that produce a personal disposition that is outgoing, sociable and demonstrative, as contrasted to being shy, restricted and inhibited.

b 1261   Agreeableness
Mental functions that produce a personal disposition that is cooperative, amicable, and accommodating, as contrasted to being unfriendly, oppositional and defiant.

b 1262   Conscientiousness
Mental functions that produce personal dispositions such as in being hard-working, methodical and scrupulous, as contrasted to mental

functions producing dispositions such as in being lazy, unreliable and irresponsible.

b 1263 Psychic stability
Mental functions that produce a personal disposition that is even-tempered, calm and composed, as contrasted to being irritable, worried, erratic and moody.

b 1264 Openness to experience
Mental functions that produce a personal disposition that is curious, imaginative, inquisitive and experience-seeking, as contrasted to being stagnant, inattentive and emotionally inexpressive.

b 1265 Optimism
Mental functions that produce a personal disposition that is cheerful, buoyant and hopeful, as contrasted to being downhearted, gloomy and despairing.

b 1266 Confidence
Mental functions that produce a personal disposition that is self-assured, bold and assertive, as contrasted to being timid, insecure and self-effacing.

b 1267 Trustworthiness
Mental functions that produce a personal disposition that is dependable and principled, as contrasted to being deceitful and antisocial.

b 1268 Temperament and personality functions, other specified

b 1269 Temperament and personality functions, unspecified

b 130 Energy and drive functions
General mental functions of physiological and psychological mechanisms that cause the individual to move towards satisfying specific needs and general goals in a persistent manner.

Inclusions: functions of energy level, motivation, appetite, craving (including craving for substances that can be abused), and impulse control

Exclusions: consciousness functions (b110); temperament and personality functions (b126); sleep functions (b134); psychomotor functions (b147); emotional functions (b152)

b 1300 Energy level
Mental functions that produce vigour and stamina.

b 1301   Motivation
Mental functions that produce the incentive to act; the conscious or unconscious driving force for action.

b 1302   Appetite
Mental functions that produce a natural longing or desire, especially the natural and recurring desire for food and drink.

b 1303   Craving
Mental functions that produce the urge to consume substances, including substances that can be abused.

b 1304   Impulse control
Mental functions that regulate and resist sudden intense urges to do something.

b 1308   Energy and drive functions, other specified

b 1309   Energy and drive functions, unspecified

b 134   Sleep functions
General mental functions of periodic, reversible and selective physical and mental disengagement from one's immediate environment accompanied by characteristic physiological changes.

Inclusions: functions of amount of sleeping, and onset, maintenance and quality of sleep; functions involving the sleep cycle, such as in insomnia, hypersomnia and narcolepsy

Exclusions: consciousness functions (b110); energy and drive functions (b130); attention functions (b140); psychomotor functions (b147)

b 1340   Amount of sleep
Mental functions involved in the time spent in the state of sleep in the diurnal cycle or circadian rhythm.

b 1341   Onset of sleep
Mental functions that produce the transition between wakefulness and sleep.

b 1342   Maintenance of sleep
Mental functions that sustain the state of being asleep.

b 1343   Quality of sleep
Mental functions that produce the natural sleep leading to optimal physical and mental rest and relaxation.

b 1344   Functions involving the sleep cycle
Mental functions that produce rapid eye movement (REM) sleep (associated with dreaming) and non-rapid eye movement sleep (NREM) (characterized by the traditional concept of sleep as a time of decreased physiological and psychological activity).

b 1348   Sleep functions, other specified

b 1349   Sleep functions, unspecified

b 139   Global mental functions, other specified and unspecified

Specific mental functions (b140-b189)

b 140   Attention functions
Specific mental functions of focusing on an external stimulus or internal experience for the required period of time.

Inclusions: functions of sustaining attention, shifting attention, dividing attention, sharing attention; concentration; distractibility

Exclusions: consciousness functions (b110); energy and drive functions (b130); sleep functions (b134); memory functions (b144); psychomotor functions (b147); perceptual functions (b156)

b 1400   Sustaining attention
Mental functions that produce concentration for the period of time required.

b 1401   Shifting attention
Mental functions that permit refocusing concentration from one stimulus to another.

b 1402   Dividing attention
Mental functions that permit focusing on two or more stimuli at the same time.

b 1403   Sharing attention
Mental functions that permit focusing on the same stimulus by two or more people, such as a child and a caregiver both focusing on a toy.

b 1408   Attention functions, other specified

b 1409   Attention functions, unspecified

b 144   Memory functions
Specific mental functions of registering and storing information and retrieving it as needed.

Inclusions: functions of short-term and long-term memory, immediate, recent and remote memory; memory span; retrieval of memory; remembering; functions used in recalling and learning, such as in nominal, selective and dissociative amnesia

Exclusions: consciousness functions (b110); orientation functions (b114); intellectual functions (b117); attention functions (b140); perceptual functions (b156); thought functions (b160); higher-level cognitive functions (b164); mental functions of language (b167); calculation functions (b172)

b 1440   Short-term memory
Mental functions that produce a temporary, disruptable memory store of around 30 seconds duration from which information is lost if not consolidated into long-term memory.

b 1441   Long-term memory
Mental functions that produce a memory system permitting the long-term storage of information from short-term memory and both autobiographical memory for past events and semantic memory for language and facts.

b 1442   Retrieval and processing of memory
Specific mental functions of recalling information stored in long-term memory and bringing it into awareness.

b 1448   Memory functions, other specified

b 1449   Memory functions, unspecified

b 147   Psychomotor functions
Specific mental functions of control over both motor and psychological events at the body level.

Inclusions: manual and lateral dominance functions of psychomotor control, such as in psychomotor delay, excitement and agitation, posturing, stereotypes, motor perseveration, catatonia, negativism, ambitendency, echopraxia and echolalia; quality of psychomotor function.

Exclusions: consciousness functions (b110); orientation functions (b114); intellectual functions (b117); energy and drive functions (b130); attention functions (b140); basic cognitive functions (b163); mental functions of language (b167); clumsiness (b760)

b 1470   Psychomotor control
Mental functions that regulate the speed of behaviour or response time that involves both motor and psychological components, such as in disruption of control producing psychomotor retardation (moving and speaking slowly; decrease in gesturing and spontaneity) or psychomotor excitement (excessive behavioural and cognitive activity, usually nonproductive and often in response to inner tension as in toe-tapping, hand-wringing, agitation, or restlessness.)

b 1471   Quality of psychomotor functions
Mental functions that produce nonverbal behaviour in the proper sequence and character of its subcomponents, such as hand and eye coordination, or gait.

b 1472   Organization of psychomotor functions
Mental functions that produce complex goal directed sequences of movement.

b 1473   Manual dominance
Development and preference in hand use.

b 1474   Lateral dominance
Development and preference of eye, and limb use.

b 1478   Psychomotor functions, other specified

b 1479   Psychomotor functions, unspecified

b 152   Emotional functions
Specific mental functions related to the feeling and affective components of the processes of the mind.

Inclusions: functions of appropriateness of emotion, regulation and range of emotion; affect; sadness, happiness, love, fear, anger, hate, tension, anxiety, joy, sorrow; lability of emotion; flattening of affect

Exclusions: temperament and personality functions (b126); energy and drive functions (b130)

b 1520   Appropriateness of emotion
Mental functions that produce congruence of feeling or affect with the situation, such as happiness at receiving good news.

b 1521   Regulation of emotion
Mental functions that control the experience and display of affect.

b 1522   Range of emotion
Mental functions that produce the spectrum of experience of arousal of affect or feelings such as love, hate, anxiousness, sorrow, joy, fear and anger.

b 1528   Emotional functions, other specified

b 1529   Emotional functions, unspecified

b 156   Perceptual functions
Specific mental functions of recognizing and interpreting sensory stimuli.

Inclusions: functions of auditory, visual, olfactory, gustatory, tactile and visuospatial perception, such as hallucination or illusion

Exclusions: consciousness functions (b110); orientation functions (b114); attention functions (b140); memory functions (b144); mental functions of language (b167); seeing and related functions (b210-b229); hearing and vestibular functions (b230-b249); additional sensory functions (b250-b279)

b 1560   Auditory perception
Mental functions involved in discriminating sounds, tones, pitches and other acoustic stimuli.

b 1561   Visual perception
Mental functions involved in discriminating shape, size, colour and other ocular stimuli.

b 1562   Olfactory perception
Mental functions involved in distinguishing differences in smells.

b 1563   Gustatory perception
Mental functions involved in distinguishing differences in tastes, such as sweet, sour, salty and bitter stimuli, detected by the tongue.

b 1564   Tactile perception
Mental functions involved in distinguishing differences in texture, such as rough or smooth stimuli, detected by touch.

b 1565   Visuospatial perception
Mental function involved in distinguishing by sight the relative position of objects in the environment or in relation to oneself.

b 1568   Perceptual functions, other specified

b 1569   Perceptual functions, unspecified

b 160   Thought functions
Specific mental functions related to the ideational component of the mind.

Inclusions: functions of pace, form, control and content of thought; goal-directed thought functions, non-goal directed thought functions; logical thought functions, such as pressure of thought, flight of ideas, thought block, incoherence of thought, tangentiality, circumstantiality, delusions, obsessions and compulsions

Exclusions: intellectual functions (b117); memory functions (b144); psychomotor functions (b147); perceptual functions (b156); higher-level cognitive functions (b164); mental functions of language (b167); calculation functions (b172)

b 1600   Pace of thought
Mental functions that govern speed of the thinking process.

b 1601   Form of thought
Mental functions that organize the thinking process as to its coherence and logic.

Inclusions: impairments of ideational perseveration, tangentiality and circumstantiality

b 1602   Content of thought
Mental functions consisting of the ideas that are present in the thinking process and what is being conceptualized.

Inclusions: impairments of delusions, overvalued ideas and somatization

b 1603   Control of thought
Mental functions that provide volitional control of thinking and are recognized as such by the person.

Inclusions: impairments of rumination, obsession, thought broadcast and thought insertion

b 1608   Thought functions, other specified

b 1609   Thought functions, unspecified

b 163   Basic cognitive functions
Mental functions involved in acquisition of knowledge about objects, events and experiences; and the organization and application of that knowledge in tasks requiring mental activity.

Inclusion: functions of cognitive development of representation, knowing and reasoning

Exclusion: higher level cognitive functions (b164)

b 164   **Higher-level cognitive functions**
Specific mental functions especially dependent on the frontal lobes of the brain, including complex goal-directed behaviours such as decision-making, abstract thinking, planning and carrying out plans, mental flexibility, and deciding which behaviours are appropriate under what circumstances; often called executive functions.

Inclusions: functions of abstraction and organization of ideas; time management, insight and judgement; concept formation, categorization and cognitive flexibility

Exclusions: memory functions (b144); thought functions (b160); mental functions of language (b167); calculation functions (b172)

> **b 1640**   **Abstraction**
> Mental functions of creating general ideas, qualities or characteristics out of, and distinct from, concrete realities, specific objects or actual instances.

> **b 1641**   **Organization and planning**
> Mental functions of coordinating parts into a whole, of systematizing; the mental function involved in developing a method of proceeding or acting.

> **b 1642**   **Time management**
> Mental functions of ordering events in chronological sequence, allocating amounts of time to events and activities.

> **b 1643**   **Cognitive flexibility**
> Mental functions of changing strategies, or shifting mental sets, especially as involved in problem-solving.

> **b 1644**   **Insight**
> Mental functions of awareness and understanding of oneself and one's behaviour.

> **b 1645**   **Judgement**
> Mental functions involved in discriminating between and evaluating different options, such as those involved in forming an opinion.

> **b 1646**   **Problem-solving**
> Mental functions of identifying, analysing and integrating incongruent or conflicting information into a solution.

b 1648　　Higher-level cognitive functions, other specified

b 1649　　Higher-level cognitive functions, unspecified

b 167　Mental functions of language
Specific mental functions of recognizing and using signs, symbols and other components of a language.

Inclusions: functions of reception and decryption of spoken, written or other forms of language such as sign language; functions of expression of spoken, written or other forms of language; integrative language functions, spoken and written, such as involved in receptive, expressive, Broca's, Wernicke's and conduction aphasia

Exclusions: attention functions (b140); memory functions (b144); perceptual functions (b156); thought functions (b160); higher-level cognitive functions (b164); calculation functions (b172); mental functions of complex movements (b176); Chapter 2 Sensory Functions and Pain; Chapter 3 Voice and Speech Functions

b 1670　　Reception of language
Specific mental functions of decoding messages in spoken, written or other forms, such as sign language, to obtain their meaning.

b 16700　　Reception of spoken language
Mental functions of decoding spoken messages to obtain their meaning.

b 16701　　Reception of written language
Mental functions of decoding written messages to obtain their meaning.

b 16702　　Reception of sign language
Mental functions of decoding messages in languages that use signs made by hands and other movements, in order to obtain their meaning.

b 16703　　Reception of gestural language
Mental functions of decoding messages in non-formalized gestures made by hands and other movements in order to obtain their meaning.

b 16708　　Reception of language, other specified

b 16709　　Reception of language, unspecified

b 1671   Expression of language
Specific mental functions necessary to produce meaningful messages in spoken, written, signed or other forms of language.

b 16710   Expression of spoken language
Mental functions necessary to produce meaningful spoken messages.

b 16711   Expression of written language
Mental functions necessary to produce meaningful written messages.

b 16712   Expression of sign language
Mental functions necessary to produce meaningful messages in languages that use signs made by hands and other movements.

b 16713   Expression of gestural language
Mental functions necessary to produce messages in non-formalized gestures made by hands and other movements.

b 16718   Expression of language, other specified

b 16719   Expression of language, unspecified

b 1672   Integrative language functions
Mental functions that organize semantic and symbolic meaning, grammatical structure and ideas for the production of messages in spoken, written or other forms of language.

b 1678   Mental functions of language, other specified

b 1679   Mental functions of language, unspecified

b 172   **Calculation functions**
Specific mental functions of determination, approximation and manipulation of mathematical symbols and processes.

Inclusions: functions of addition, subtraction, and other simple mathematical calculations; functions of complex mathematical operations

Exclusions: attention functions (b140); memory functions (b144); thought functions (b160); higher-level cognitive functions (b164); mental functions of language (b167)

b 1720 Simple calculation
Mental functions of computing with numbers, such as addition, subtraction, multiplication and division.

b 1721 Complex calculation
Mental functions of translating word problems into arithmetic procedures, translating mathematical formulas into arithmetic procedures, and other complex manipulations involving numbers.

b 1728 Calculation functions, other specified

b 1729 Calculation functions, unspecified

b 176 Mental function of sequencing complex movements
Specific mental functions of sequencing and coordinating complex, purposeful movements.

Inclusions: impairments such as in ideation, ideomotor, dressing, oculomotor and speech apraxia

Exclusions: psychomotor functions (b147); higher-level cognitive functions (b164); Chapter 7 Neuromusculoskeletal and Movement-Related Functions

b 180 Experience of self and time functions
Specific mental functions related to the awareness of one's identity, one's body, one's position in the reality of one's environment and of time.

Inclusions: functions of experience of self, body image and time

b 1800 Experience of self
Specific mental functions of being aware of one's own identity and one's position in the reality of the environment around oneself.

Inclusion: impairments such as depersonalization and derealization

b 1801 Body image
Specific mental functions related to the representation and awareness of one's body.

Inclusion: impairments such as phantom limb and feeling too fat or too thin

b 1802 Experience of time
Specific mental functions of the subjective experiences related to the length and passage of time.

Inclusion: impairments such as jamais vu and déjà vu

      b 1808   Experience of self and time functions, other specified

      b 1809   Experience of self and time functions, unspecified

b 189   Specific mental functions, other specified and unspecified

b 198   Mental functions, other specified

b 199   Mental functions, unspecified

Chapter 2

Sensory functions and pain

This chapter is about the functions of the senses, seeing, hearing, tasting and so on, as well as the sensation of pain.

Seeing and related functions (b210-b229)

b 210   **Seeing functions**
Sensory functions relating to sensing the presence of light and sensing the form, size, shape and colour of the visual stimuli.

Inclusions: visual acuity functions; visual field functions; quality of vision; functions of sensing light and colour, visual acuity of distant and near vision, monocular and binocular vision; visual picture quality; impairments such as myopia, hypermetropia, astigmatism, hemianopia, colour-blindness, tunnel vision, central and peripheral scotoma, diplopia, night blindness and impaired adaptability to light

Exclusion: perceptual functions (b156)

b 2100   Visual acuity functions
Seeing functions of sensing form and contour, both binocular and monocular, for both distant and near vision.

b 21000   Binocular acuity of distant vision
Seeing functions of sensing size, form and contour, using both eyes, for objects distant from the eye.

b 21001   Monocular acuity of distant vision
Seeing functions of sensing size, form and contour, using either right or left eye alone, for objects distant from the eye.

b 21002   Binocular acuity of near vision
Seeing functions of sensing size, form and contour, using both eyes, for objects close to the eye.

b 21003   Monocular acuity of near vision
Seeing functions of sensing size, form and contour, using either right or left eye alone, for objects close to the eye.

b 21008   Visual acuity functions, other specified

b 21009   Visual acuity functions, unspecified

b 2101   **Visual field functions**
Seeing functions related to the entire area that can be seen with fixation of gaze.

Inclusions: impairments such as in scotoma, tunnel vision, anopsia

b 2102   **Quality of vision**
Seeing functions involving light sensitivity, colour vision, contrast sensitivity and the overall quality of the picture.

b 21020   **Light sensitivity**
Seeing functions of sensing a minimum amount of light (light minimum), and the minimum difference in intensity (light difference.)

Inclusions: functions of dark adaptation; impairments, such as night blindness (hyposensitivity to light) and photophobia (hypersensitivity to light)

b 21021   **Colour vision**
Seeing functions of differentiating and matching colours.

b 21022   **Contrast sensitivity**
Seeing functions of separating figure from ground, involving the minimum amount of luminance required.

b 21023   **Visual picture quality**
Seeing functions involving the quality of the picture.

Inclusions: impairments such as in seeing stray lights, affected picture quality (floaters or webbing), picture distortion, and seeing stars or flashes

b 21028   **Quality of vision, other specified**

b 21029   **Quality of vision, unspecified**

b 2108   **Seeing functions, other specified**

b 2109   **Seeing functions, unspecified**

b 215   **Functions of structures adjoining the eye**
Functions of structures in and around the eye that facilitate seeing functions.

Inclusions: functions of internal muscles of the eye, eyelid, external muscles of the eye, including voluntary and tracking movements and fixation of the eye, lachrymal glands, accommodation, pupillary reflex; impairments such as in nystagmus, xerophthalmia and ptosis

Exclusions: seeing functions (b210); Chapter 7 Neuromusculoskeletal and Movement-related Functions

b 2150 Functions of internal muscles of the eye
Functions of the muscles inside the eye, such as the iris, that adjust the shape and size of the pupil and lens of the eye.

Inclusions: functions of accommodation; pupillary reflex

b 2151 Functions of the eyelid
Functions of the eyelid, such as the protective reflex.

b 2152 Functions of external muscles of the eye
Functions of the muscles that are used to look in different directions, to follow an object as it moves across the visual field, to produce saccadic jumps to catch up with a moving target, and to fix the eye.

Inclusions: nystagmus; cooperation of both eyes

b 2153 Functions of lachrymal glands
Functions of the tear glands and ducts.

b 2158 Functions of structures adjoining the eye, other specified

b 2159 Functions of structures adjoining the eye, unspecified

b 220 Sensations associated with the eye and adjoining structures
Sensations of tired, dry and itching eye and related feelings.

Inclusions: feelings of pressure behind the eye, of something in the eye, eye strain, burning in the eye; eye irritation

Exclusion: sensation of pain (b280)

b 229 Seeing and related functions, other specified and unspecified

Hearing and vestibular functions (b230-b249)

b 230 **Hearing functions**
Sensory functions relating to sensing the presence of sounds and discriminating the location, pitch, loudness and quality of sounds.

Inclusions: functions of hearing, auditory discrimination, localization of sound source, lateralization of sound, speech discrimination; impairments such as deafness, hearing impairment and hearing loss

Exclusions: perceptual functions (b156) and mental functions of language (b167)

b 2300 **Sound detection**
Sensory functions relating to sensing the presence of sounds.

b 2301 **Sound discrimination**
Sensory functions relating to sensing the presence of sound involving the differentiation of ground and binaural synthesis, separation and blending.

b 2302 **Localisation of sound source**
Sensory functions relating to determining the location of the source of sound.

b 2303 **Lateralization of sound**
Sensory functions relating to determining whether the sound is coming from the right or left side.

b 2304 **Speech discrimination**
Sensory functions relating to determining spoken language and distinguishing it from other sounds.

b 2308 **Hearing functions, other specified**

b 2309 **Hearing functions, unspecified**

b 235 **Vestibular functions**
Sensory functions of the inner ear related to position, balance and movement.

Inclusions: functions of position and positional sense; functions of balance of the body and movement

Exclusion: sensation associated with hearing and vestibular functions (b240)

b 2350   **Vestibular function of position**
Sensory functions of the inner ear related to determining the position of the body.

b 2351   **Vestibular function of balance**
Sensory functions of the inner ear related to determining the balance of the body.

b 2352   **Vestibular function of determination of movement**
Sensory functions of the inner ear related to determining movement of the body, including its direction and speed.

b 2358   **Vestibular functions, other specified**

b 2359   **Vestibular functions, unspecified**

b 240   **Sensations associated with hearing and vestibular function**
Sensations of dizziness, falling, tinnitus and vertigo.

Inclusions: sensations of ringing in ears, irritation in ear, aural pressure, nausea associated with dizziness or vertigo

Exclusions: vestibular functions (b235); sensation of pain (b280)

b 2400   **Ringing in ears or tinnitus**
Sensation of low-pitched rushing, hissing or ringing in the ear.

b 2401   **Dizziness**
Sensation of motion involving either oneself or one's environment; sensation of rotating, swaying or tilting.

b 2402   **Sensation of falling**
Sensation of losing one's grip and falling.

b 2403   **Nausea associated with dizziness or vertigo**
Sensation of wanting to vomit that arises from dizziness or vertigo.

b 2404   **Irritation in the ear**
Sensation of itching or other similar sensations in the ear.

b 2405   **Aural pressure**
Sensation of pressure in the ear.

b 2408   Sensations associated with hearing and vestibular function, other specified

b 2409   Sensations associated with hearing and vestibular function, unspecified

b 249   Hearing and vestibular functions, other specified and unspecified

Additional sensory functions (b250-b279)

b 250   Taste function
Sensory functions of sensing qualities of bitterness, sweetness, sourness and saltiness.

Inclusions: gustatory functions; impairments such as ageusia and hypogeusia

b 255   Smell function
Sensory functions of sensing odours and smells.

Inclusions: olfactory functions; impairments such as anosmia or hyposmia

b 260   Proprioceptive function
Sensory functions of sensing the relative position of body parts.

Inclusions: functions of statesthesia and kinaesthesia

Exclusions: vestibular functions (b235); sensations related to muscles and movement functions (b780)

b 265   Touch function
Sensory functions of sensing surfaces and their texture or quality.

Inclusions: functions of touching, feeling of touch; impairments such as numbness, anaesthesia, tingling, paraesthesia and hyperaesthesia

Exclusions: sensory functions related to temperature and other stimuli (b270)

b 270   Sensory functions related to temperature and other stimuli
Sensory functions of sensing temperature, vibration, pressure and noxious stimulus.

Inclusions: functions of being sensitive to temperature, vibration, shaking or oscillation, superficial pressure, deep pressure, burning sensation or a noxious stimulus

Exclusions: touch functions (b265); sensation of pain (b280)

b 2700 **Sensitivity to temperature**
Sensory functions of sensing cold and heat.

b 2701 **Sensitivity to vibration**
Sensory functions of sensing shaking or oscillation.

b 2702 **Sensitivity to pressure**
Sensory functions of sensing pressure against or on the skin.

Inclusions: impairments such as sensitivity to touch, numbness, hypaesthesia, hyperaesthesia, paraesthesia and tingling

b 2703 **Sensitivity to a noxious stimulus**
Sensory functions of sensing painful or uncomfortable sensations.

Inclusions: impairments such as hypalgesia, hyperpathia, allodynia, analgesia and anaesthesia dolorosa

b 2708 **Sensory functions related to temperature and other stimuli, other specified**

b 2709 **Sensory functions related to temperature and other stimuli, unspecified**

b 279 **Additional sensory functions, other specified and unspecified**

Pain (b280-b289)

b 280 **Sensation of pain**
Sensation of unpleasant feeling indicating potential or actual damage to some body structure.

Inclusions: sensations of generalized or localized pain, in one or more body part, pain in a dermatome, stabbing pain, burning pain, dull pain, aching pain; impairments such as myalgia, analgesia and hyperalgesia

b 2800 **Generalized pain**
Sensation of unpleasant feeling indicating potential or actual damage to some body structure felt all over, or throughout the body.

b 2801 **Pain in body part**
Sensation of unpleasant feeling indicating potential or actual damage to some body structure felt in a specific part, or parts, of the body.

b 28010   Pain in head and neck
Sensation of unpleasant feeling indicating potential or actual damage to some body structure felt in the head and neck.

b 28011   Pain in chest
Sensation of unpleasant feeling indicating potential or actual damage to some body structure felt in the chest.

b 28012   Pain in stomach or abdomen
Sensation of unpleasant feeling indicating potential or actual damage to some body structure felt in the stomach or abdomen.

Inclusion: pain in the pelvic region

b 28013   Pain in back
Sensation of unpleasant feeling indicating potential or actual damage to some body structure felt in the back.

Inclusions: pain in the trunk; low backache

b 28014   Pain in upper limb
Sensation of unpleasant feeling indicating potential or actual damage to some body structure felt in either one or both upper limbs, including hands.

b 28015   Pain in lower limb
Sensation of unpleasant feeling indicating potential or actual damage to some body structure felt in either one or both lower limbs, including feet.

b 28016   Pain in joints
Sensation of unpleasant feeling indicating potential or actual damage to some body structure felt in one or more joints, including small and big joints.

Inclusions: pain in the hip; pain in the shoulder

b 28018   Pain in body part, other specified

b 28019   Pain in body part, unspecified

b 2802   Pain in multiple body parts
Unpleasant sensation indicating potential or actual damage to some body structure located in several body parts.

b 2803 Radiating pain in a dermatome
Unpleasant sensation indicating potential or actual damage to some body structure located in areas of skin served by the same nerve root.

b 2804 Radiating pain in a segment or region
Unpleasant sensation indicating potential or actual damage to some body structure located in areas of skin in different body parts not served by the same nerve root.

b 289 Sensation of pain, other specified and unspecified

b 298 Sensory functions and pain, other specified

b 299 Sensory functions and pain, unspecified

Chapter 3

Voice and speech functions

This chapter is about the functions of producing sounds and speech.

b 310   **Voice functions**
Functions of the production of various sounds by the passage of air through the larynx.
Inclusions: functions of production and quality of voice; functions of phonation, pitch, loudness and other qualities of voice; impairments such as aphonia, dysphonia, hoarseness, hypernasality and hyponasality

Exclusions: mental functions of language (b167); articulation functions (b320); babbling (b3401)

> **b 3100**   **Production of voice**
> Functions of the production of sound made through coordination of the larynx and surrounding muscles with the respiratory system.
>
> *Inclusions: functions of phonation, loudness; impairment of aphonia*

> **b 3101**   **Quality of voice**
> Functions of the production of characteristics of voice including pitch, resonance and other features.
>
> *Inclusions: functions of high or low pitch; impairments such as hypernasality, hyponasality, dysphonia, hoarseness or harshness*

> **b 3108**   **Voice functions, other specified**

> **b 3109**   **Voice functions, unspecified**

b 320   **Articulation functions**
Functions of the production of speech sounds.

Inclusions: functions of enunciation, articulation of phonemes; spastic, ataxic, flaccid dysarthria; anarthria

Exclusions: mental functions of language (b167); voice functions (b310)

b 330   **Fluency and rhythm of speech functions**
Functions of the production of flow and tempo of speech.

Inclusions: functions of fluency, rhythm, speed and melody of speech; prosody and intonation; impairments such as stuttering, stammering, cluttering, bradylalia and tachylalia

Exclusions: mental functions of language (b167); voice functions (b310); articulation functions (b320)

b 3300   **Fluency of speech**

Functions of the production of smooth, uninterrupted flow of speech.

Inclusions: functions of smooth connection of speech; impairments such as stuttering, stammering, cluttering, dysfluency, repetition of sounds, words or parts of words and irregular breaks in speech

b 3301   **Rhythm of speech**

Functions of the modulated, tempo and stress patterns in speech.

Inclusions: impairments such as stereotypic or repetitive speech cadence

b 3302   **Speed of speech**

Functions of the rate of speech production.

Inclusions: impairments such as bradylalia and tachylalia

b 3303   **Melody of speech**

Functions of modulation of pitch patterns in speech.

Inclusions: prosody of speech, intonation, melody of speech; impairments such as monotone speech

b 3308   **Fluency and rhythm of speech functions, other specified**

b 3309   **Fluency and rhythm of speech functions, unspecified**

b 340   **Alternative vocalization functions**

Functions of the production of other manners of vocalization.

Inclusions: functions of the production of notes and range of sounds, such as in singing, chanting, babbling and humming; crying aloud and screaming

Exclusions: mental functions of language (b167); voice functions (b310); articulation functions (b320); fluency and rhythm of speech functions (b330)

b 3400   **Production of notes**

Functions of production of musical vocal sounds.

Inclusions: sustaining, modulating and terminating production of single or connected vocalizations with variation in pitch such as in singing, humming and chanting

b 3401   Making a range of sounds
Functions of production of a variety of vocalizations.

Inclusions: functions of crying, cooing, gurgling and babbling

b 3408   Alternative vocalization functions, other specified

b 3409   Alternative vocalization functions, unspecified

b 398   Voice and speech functions, other specified

b 399   Voice and speech functions, unspecified

Chapter 4

Functions of the cardiovascular, haematological, immunological and respiratory systems

This chapter is about the functions involved in the cardiovascular system (functions of the heart and blood vessels), the haematological and immunological systems (functions of blood production and immunity), and the respiratory system (functions of respiration and exercise tolerance).

Functions of the cardiovascular system (b410-b429)

b 410 **Heart functions**
Functions of pumping the blood in adequate or required amounts and pressure throughout the body.

Inclusions: functions of heart rate, rhythm and output; contraction force of ventricular muscles; functions of heart valves; pumping the blood through the pulmonary circuit; dynamics of circulation to the heart; impairments such as tachycardia, bradycardia and irregular heart beatand as in heart failure, cardiomyopathy, myocarditis,and coronary insufficiency

Exclusions: blood vessel functions (b415); blood pressure functions (b420); exercise tolerance functions (b455)

    b 4100 **Heart rate**
Functions related to the number of times the heart contracts every minute.

Inclusions: impairments such as rates that are too fast (tachycardia) or too slow (bradycardia)

    b 4101 **Heart rhythm**
Functions related to the regularity of the beating of the heart.

Inclusions: impairments such as arrhythmias

    b 4102 **Contraction force of ventricular muscles**
Functions related to the amount of blood pumped by the ventricular muscles during every beat.

Inclusions: impairments such as diminished cardiac output

    b 4103 **Blood supply to the heart**
Functions related to the volume of blood available to the heart muscle.

Inclusion: impairments such as coronary ischaemia

b 4108   Heart functions, other specified

b 4109   Heart functions, unspecified

b 415   Blood vessel functions
Functions of transporting blood throughout the body.

Inclusions: functions of arteries, capillaries and veins; vasomotor function; functions of pulmonary arteries, capillaries and veins; functions of valves of veins; impairments such as in blockage or constriction of arteries; atherosclerosis, arteriosclerosis, thromboembolism and varicose veins

Exclusions: heart functions (b410); blood pressure functions (b420); haematological system functions (b430); exercise tolerance functions (b455)

b 4150   Functions of arteries
functions related to blood flow in the arteries

Inclusions: impairments such as arterial dilation; arterial constriction such as in intermittent claudication

b 4151   Functions of capillaries
Functions related to blood flow in the capillaries.

b 4152   Functions of veins
Functions related to blood flow in the veins, and the functions of valves of veins.

Inclusions: impairments such as venous dilation; venous constriction; insufficient closing of valves as in varicose veins

b 4158   Blood vessel functions, other specified

b 4159   Blood vessel functions, unspecified

b 420   Blood pressure functions
Functions of maintaining the pressure of blood within the arteries.

Inclusions: functions of maintenance of blood pressure; increased and decreased blood pressure; impairments such as in hypotension, hypertension and postural hypotension

Exclusions: heart functions (b410); blood vessel functions (b415); exercise tolerance functions (b455)

b 4200   **Increased blood pressure**
Functions related to a rise in systolic or diastolic blood pressure above normal for the age.

b 4201   **Decreased blood pressure**
Functions related to a fall in systolic or diastolic blood pressure below normal for the age.

b 4202   **Maintenance of blood pressure**
Functions related to maintaining an appropriate blood pressure in response to changes in the body.

b 4208   **Blood pressure functions, other specified**

b 4209   **Blood pressure functions, unspecified**

b 429   Functions of the cardiovascular system, other specified and unspecified

Functions of the haematological and immunological systems (b430-b439)

b 430   Haematological system functions
Functions of blood production, oxygen and metabolite carriage, and clotting.

Inclusions: functions of the production of blood and bone marrow; oxygen-carrying functions of blood; blood-related functions of spleen; metabolite-carrying functions of blood; clotting; impairments such as anaemia, haemophilia and other clotting dysfunctions

Exclusions: functions of the cardiovascular system (b410-b429); immunological system functions (b435); exercise tolerance functions (b455)

b 4300   **Production of blood**
Functions related to the production of blood and all its constituents.

b 4301   **Oxygen-carrying functions of the blood**
Functions related to the blood's capacity to carry oxygen throughout the body.

b 4302   **Metabolite-carrying functions of the blood**
Functions related to the blood's capacity to carry metabolites throughout the body.

b 4303   **Clotting functions**
Functions related to the coagulation of blood, such as at a site of injury.

b 4308   Haematological system functions, other specified

b 4309   Haematological system functions, unspecified

b 435   Immunological system functions
Functions of the body related to protection against foreign substances, including infections, by specific and non-specific immune responses.

Inclusions: immune response (specific and non-specific); hypersensitivity reactions; functions of lymphatic vessels and nodes; functions of cell-mediated immunity, antibody-mediated immunity; response to immunization; impairments such as in autoimmunity, allergic reactions, lymphadenitis and lymphoedema

Exclusion: haematological system functions (b430)

b 4350   Immune response
Functions of the body's response of sensitization to foreign substances, including infections.

b 43500   Specific immune response
Functions of the body's response of sensitization to a specific foreign substance.

b 43501   Non-specific immune response
Functions of the body's general response of sensitization to foreign substances, including infections.

b 43508   Immune response, other specified

b 43509   Immune response, unspecified

b 4351   Hypersensitivity reactions
Functions of the body's response of increased sensitization to foreign substances, such as in sensitivities to different antigens.

Inclusions: impairments such as hypersensitivities or allergies

Exclusion: tolerance to food (b5153)

b 4352   Functions of lymphatic vessels
Functions related to vascular channels that transport lymph.

b 4353   Functions of lymph nodes
Functions related to glands along the course of lymphatic vessels.

b 4358   Immunological system functions, other specified

b 4359   Immunological system functions, unspecified

b 439   Functions of the haematological and immunological systems, other specified and unspecified

Functions of the respiratory system (b440-b449)

b 440   Respiration functions
Functions of inhaling air into the lungs, the exchange of gases between air and blood, and exhaling air.

Inclusions: functions of respiration rate, rhythm and depth; impairments such as apnoea, hyperventilation, irregular respiration, paradoxical respiration, and bronchial spasm, and as in pulmonary emphysema; upper pulmonary obstruction, reduction in airflow through upper and lower airways

Exclusions: respiratory muscle functions (b445); additional respiratory functions (b450); exercise tolerance functions (b455)

b 4400   Respiration rate
Functions related to the number of breaths taken per minute.

Inclusions: impairments such as rates that are too fast (tachypnoea) or too slow (bradypnoea)

b 4401   Respiratory rhythm
Functions related to the periodicity and regularity of breathing.

Inclusions: impairments such as irregular breathing

b 4402   Depth of respiration
Functions related to the volume of expansion of the lungs during breathing.

Inclusions: impairments such as superficial or shallow respiration

b 4408   Respiration functions, other specified

b 4409   Respiration functions, unspecified

b 445   Respiratory muscle functions
Functions of the muscles involved in breathing.

Inclusions: functions of thoracic respiratory muscles; functions of the diaphragm; functions of accessory respiratory muscles

Exclusions: respiration functions (b440); additional respiratory functions (b450); exercise tolerance functions (b455)

b 4450   Functions of the thoracic respiratory muscles
Functions of the thoracic muscles involved in breathing.

b 4451   Functions of the diaphragm
Functions of the diaphragm as involved in breathing.

b 4452   Functions of accessory respiratory muscles
Functions of the additional muscles involved in breathing.

b 4458   Respiratory muscle functions, other specified

b 4459   Respiratory muscle functions, unspecified

b 449   Functions of the respiratory system, other specified and unspecified

Additional functions and sensations of the cardiovascular and respiratory systems (b450-b469)

b 450   **Additional respiratory functions**
Additional functions related to breathing, such as coughing, sneezing and yawning.

Inclusions: functions of blowing, whistling and mouth breathing, functions of producing and transporting mucus

b 4500   Production of airway mucus
Functions of producing mucus of upper and lower airways.

b 4501   Transportation of airways mucus
Functions of transporting mucus of upper and lower airways.

b 4508   Additional respiratory functions, other specified

b 4509   Additional respiratory functions, unspecified

b 455   **Exercise tolerance functions**
Functions related to respiratory and cardiovascular capacity as required for enduring physical exertion.

Inclusions: functions of physical endurance, aerobic capacity, stamina and fatiguability

Exclusions: functions of the cardiovascular system (b410-b429); haematological system functions (b430); respiration functions (b440); respiratory muscle functions (b445); additional respiratory functions (b450)

b 4550   General physical endurance
Functions related to the general level of tolerance of physical exercise or stamina.

b 4551   Aerobic capacity
Functions related to the extent to which a person can exercise without getting out of breath.

b 4552   Fatiguability
Functions related to susceptibility to fatigue, at any level of exertion.

b 4558   Exercise tolerance functions, other specified

b 4559   Exercise tolerance functions, unspecified

b 460   **Sensations associated with cardiovascular and respiratory functions**
Sensations such as missing a heart beat, palpitation and shortness of breath.

Inclusions: sensations of tightness of chest, feelings of irregular beat, dyspnoea, air hunger, choking, gagging and wheezing

Exclusion: sensation of pain (b280)

b 469   **Additional functions and sensations of the cardiovascular and respiratory systems, other specified and unspecified**

b 498   **Functions of the cardiovascular, haematological, immunological and respiratory systems, other specified**

b 499   **Functions of the cardiovascular, haematological, immunological and respiratory systems, unspecified**

Chapter 5

Functions of the digestive, metabolic and endocrine systems

This chapter is about the functions of ingestion, digestion and elimination, as well as functions involved in metabolism and the endocrine glands, and the growth maintenance functions.

Functions related to the digestive system (b510-b539)

b510 **Ingestion functions**
Functions related to taking in and manipulating solids or liquids through the mouth into the body.

Inclusions: functions of sucking, chewing and biting, manipulating food in the mouth, salivation, swallowing, burping, regurgitation, spitting and vomiting; impairments such as dysphagia, aspiration of food, aerophagia, excessive salivation, drooling and insufficient salivation

Exclusion: sensations associated with digestive system (b535)

> **b 5100** **Sucking**
> Functions of drawing into the mouth by a suction force produced by movements of the cheeks, lips and tongue.

> **b 5101** **Biting**
> Functions of cutting into, piercing or tearing off food with the front teeth.

> **b 5102** **Chewing**
> Functions of crushing, grinding and masticating food with the back teeth (e.g. molars).

> **b 5103** **Manipulation of food in the mouth**
> Functions of moving food around the mouth with the teeth and tongue.

> **b 5104** **Salivation**
> Function of the production of saliva within the mouth.

> **b 5105** **Swallowing**
> Functions of clearing the food and drink through the oral cavity, pharynx and oesophagus into the stomach at an appropriate rate and speed.
>
> *Inclusions: oral, pharyngeal or oesophageal dysphagia; impairments in oesophageal passage of food*

b 51050   **Oral swallowing**
Function of clearing the food and drink through the oral cavity at an appropriate rate and speed.

b 51051   **Pharyngeal swallowing**
Function of clearing the food and drink through the pharynx at an appropriate rate and speed.

b 51052   **Oesophageal swallowing**
Function of clearing the food and drink through the oesophagus at an appropriate rate and speed.

b 51058   **Swallowing, other specified**

b 51059   **Swallowing, unspecified**

b 5106   **Vomiting**
Functions of moving food or liquid in the reverse direction to ingestion, from stomach to oesophagus to mouth and out, such as in gastro-esophegeal reflux, recurrent vomiting, pyloric stenosis.

b 51060   **Regurgitating**
Functions of moving food or liquid in the reverse direction to ingestion, from stomach to oesophagus to mouth without expelling it.

b 5107   **Ruminating**
Functions of maintaining and manipulating vomit in the mouth.

b 5108   **Ingestion functions, other specified**

b 5109   **Ingestion functions, unspecified**

b515   **Digestive functions**
Functions of transporting food through the gastrointestinal tract, breakdown of food and absorption of nutrients.

Inclusions: functions of transport of food through the stomach, peristalsis; breakdown of food, enzyme production and action in stomach and intestines; absorption of nutrients and tolerance to food; impairments such as in hyperacidity of stomach, malabsorption, intolerance to food, hypermotility of intestines, intestinal paralysis, intestinal obstruction and decreased bile production

Exclusions: ingestion functions (b510); assimilation functions (b520); defecation functions (b525); sensations associated with the digestive system (b535)

b 5150   Transport of food through stomach and intestines
Peristalsis and related functions that mechanically move food through stomach and intestines.

b 5151   Breakdown of food
Functions of mechanically reducing food to smaller particles in the gastrointestinal tract.

b 5152   Absorption of nutrients
Functions of passing food and drink nutrients into the blood stream from along the intestines.

b 5153   Tolerance to food
Functions of accepting suitable food and drink for digestion and rejecting what is unsuitable.

Inclusion: impairments such as hypersensitivities, gluten intolerance

b 5158   Digestive functions, other specified

b 5159   Digestive functions, unspecified

b 520   Assimilation functions
Functions by which nutrients are converted into components of the living body.

Inclusion: functions of storage of nutrients in the body

Exclusions: digestive functions (b515); defecation functions (b525); weight maintenance functions (b530); general metabolic functions (b540)

b 525   Defecation functions
Functions of elimination of wastes and undigested food as faeces and related functions.

Inclusions: functions of elimination, faecal consistency, frequency of defecation; faecal continence, flatulence; impairments such as constipation, diarrhoea, watery stool and anal sphincter incompetence or incontinence

Exclusions: digestive functions (b515); assimilation functions (b520); sensations associated with the digestive system (b535)

b 5250   Elimination of faeces
Functions of the elimination of waste from the rectum, including the functions of contraction of the abdominal muscles in doing so.

b 5251 Faecal consistency
Consistency of faeces such as hard, firm, soft or watery.

b 5252 Frequency of defecation
Functions involved in the frequency of defecation.

b 5253 Faecal continence
Functions involved in voluntary control over the elimination function.

b 5254 Flatulence
Functions involved in the expulsion of excessive amounts of air or gases from the intestines.

b 5258 Defecation functions, other specified

b 5259 Defecation functions, unspecified

b 530 Weight maintenance functions
Functions of maintaining appropriate body weight, including weight gain during the developmental period.

Inclusions: functions of maintenance of acceptable Body Mass Index (BMI); and impairments such as underweight, cachexia, wasting, overweight, emaciation and such as in primary and secondary obesity

Exclusions: assimilation functions (b520); general metabolic functions (b540); endocrine gland functions (b555)

b 535 Sensations associated with the digestive system
Sensations arising from eating, drinking and related digestive functions.

Inclusions: sensations of nausea, feeling bloated, and the feeling of abdominal cramps; fullness of stomach, globus feeling, spasm of stomach, gas in stomach and heartburn

Exclusions: sensation of pain (b280); ingestion functions (b510); digestive functions (b515); defecation functions (b525)

b 5350 Sensation of nausea
Sensation of needing to vomit.

b 5351 Feeling bloated
Sensation of distension of the stomach or abdomen.

> **b 5352** **Sensation of abdominal cramp**
> Sensation of spasmodic or painful muscular contractions of the smooth muscles of the gastrointestinal tract.

> **b 5358** Sensations associated with the digestive system, other specified

> **b 5359** Sensations associated with the digestive system, unspecified

b 539 Functions related to the digestive system, other specified and unspecified

Functions related to metabolism and the endocrine system (b540-b569)

b 540 General metabolic functions
Functions of regulation of essential components of the body such as carbohydrates, proteins and fats, the conversion of one to another, and their breakdown into energy.

Inclusions: functions of metabolism, basal metabolic rate, metabolism of carbohydrate, protein and fat, catabolism, anabolism, energy production in the body; increase or decrease in metabolic rate

Exclusions: assimilation functions (b520); weight maintenance functions (b530); water, mineral and electrolyte balance functions (b545); thermoregulatory functions (b550); endocrine glands functions (b555)

> **b 5400** **Basal metabolic rate**
> Functions involved in oxygen consumption of the body at specified conditions of rest and temperature.
>
> *Inclusions: increase or decrease in basic metabolic rate; impairments such as in hyperthyroidism and hypothyroidism*

> **b 5401** **Carbohydrate metabolism**
> Functions involved in the process by which carbohydrates in the diet are stored and broken down into glucose and subsequently into carbon dioxide and water.

> **b 5402** **Protein metabolism**
> Functions involved in the process by which proteins in the diet are converted to amino acids and broken down further in the body.

> **b 5403** **Fat metabolism**
> Functions involved in the process by which fat in the diet is stored and broken down in the body.

b 5408   General metabolic functions, other specified

b 5409   General metabolic functions, unspecified

b 545   Water, mineral and electrolyte balance functions
Functions of the regulation of water, mineral and electrolytes in the body.

Inclusions: functions of water balance, balance of minerals such as calcium, zinc and iron, and balance of electrolytes such as sodium and potassium; impairments such as in water retention, dehydration, hypercalcaemia, hypocalcaemia, iron deficiency, hypernatraemia, hyponatraemia, hyperkalaemia and hypokalaemia

Exclusions: haematological system functions (b430); general metabolic functions (b540); endocrine gland functions (b555)

b 5450   Water balance
Functions involved in maintaining the level or amount of water in the body.

Inclusions: impairments such as in dehydration and rehydration

b 54500   Water retention
Functions involved in keeping water in the body.

b 54501   Maintenance of water balance
Functions involved in maintaining the optimal amount of water in the body.

b 54508   Water balance functions, other specified

b 54509   Water balance functions, unspecified

b 5451   Mineral balance
Functions involved in maintaining an equilibrium between intake, storage, utilization and excretion of minerals in the body.

b 5452   Electrolyte balance
Functions involved in maintaining an equilibrium between intake, storage, utilization and excretion of electrolytes in the body.

b 5458   Water, mineral and electrolyte balance functions, other specified

b 5459   Water, mineral and electrolyte balance functions, unspecified

b 550 **Thermoregulatory functions**
Functions of the regulation of body temperature.

Inclusions: functions of maintenance of body temperature; impairments such as hypothermia, hyperthermia

Exclusions: general metabolic functions (b540); endocrine gland functions (b555)

    b 5500 **Body temperature**
    Functions involved in regulating the core temperature of the body.

    Inclusions: impairments such as hyperthermia or hypothermia

    b 5501 **Maintenance of body temperature**
    Functions involved in maintaining optimal body temperature as environmental temperature changes.

    Inclusion: tolerance to heat or cold

    b 5508 **Thermoregulatory functions, other specified**

    b 5509 **Thermoregulatory functions, unspecified**

b 555 **Endocrine gland functions**
Functions of production and regulation of hormonal levels in the body, including cyclical changes.

Inclusions: functions of hormonal balance; hyperpituitarism, hypopituitarism, hyperthyroidism, hypothyroidism, hyperadrenalism, hypoadrenalism, hyperparathyroidism, hypoparathyroidism, hypergonadism, hypogonadism

Exclusions: general metabolic functions (b540); water, mineral and electrolyte balance functions (b545); thermoregulatory functions (b550); sexual functions (b640); menstruation functions (b650)

    b 5550 **Pubertal functions**
    Functions associated with the onset of puberty and manifestations of primary and secondary sexual characteristics.

        b 55500 **Body and pubic hair development**
        Functions associated with the development of body and pubic hair.

        b 55501 **Breast and nipple development**
        Functions associated with breast and nipple development.

           b 55502   **Penis, testes and scrotum development**
                        Functions associated with development of penis, testes and scrotum.

           b 55508   **Pubertal functions, other specified**

           b 55509   **Pubertal functions, unspecified**

b 560   **Growth maintenance functions**
Functions of attaining expected growth milestones according to contextually adjusted normative auxological parameters.

Inclusion: dwarfism and gigantism

b 569   **Functions related to metabolism and the endocrine system, other specified and unspecified**

b 598   **Functions of the digestive, metabolic and endocrine systems, other specified**

b 599   **Functions of the digestive, metabolic and endocrine systems, unspecified**

Chapter 6

Genitourinary and reproductive functions

This chapter is about the functions of urination and the reproductive functions, including sexual and procreative functions.

Urinary functions (b610-b639)

b 610   **Urinary excretory functions**
Functions of filtration and collection of the urine.

Inclusions: functions of urinary filtration, collection of urine; impairments such as in renal insufficiency, anuria, oliguria, hydronephrosis, hypotonic urinary bladder and ureteric obstruction

Exclusion: urination functions (b620)

      b 6100   **Filtration of urine**
                        Functions of filtration of urine by the kidneys.

      b 6101   **Collection of urine**
                        Functions of collection and storage of urine by the ureters and bladder.

      b 6108   **Urinary excretory functions, other specified**

      b 6109   **Urinary excretory functions, unspecified**

b 620   **Urination functions**
Functions of discharge of urine from the urinary bladder.

Inclusions: functions of urination, frequency of urination, urinary continence; impairments such as in stress, urge, reflex, overflow, continuous incontinence, dribbling, automatic bladder, polyuria, urinary retention and urinary urgency

Exclusions: urinary excretory functions (b610); sensations associated with urinary functions (b630)

         b 6200   **Urination**
                            Functions of voiding the urinary bladder.

                            Inclusions: impairments such as in urine retention

         b 6201   **Frequency of urination**
                            Functions involved in the number of times urination occurs.

      b 6202   **Urinary continence**
                Functions of control over urination.

                Inclusions:impairments such as in stress, urge, reflex, continuous and mixed incontinence

      b 6208   **Urination functions, other specified**

      b 6209   **Urination functions, unspecified**

b 630   **Sensations associated with urinary functions**
Sensations arising from voiding and related urinary functions.

Inclusions: sensations of incomplete voiding of urine, feeling of fullness of bladder

Exclusions: sensations of pain (b280); urination functions (b620)

b 639   **Urinary functions, other specified and unspecified**

Genital and reproductive functions (b640-b679)

b 640   **Sexual functions**
Mental and physical functions related to the sexual act, including the arousal, preparatory, orgasmic and resolution stages.

Inclusions: functions of the sexual arousal, preparatory, orgasmic and resolution phase: functions related to sexual interest, performance, penile erection, clitoral erection, vaginal lubrication, masturbation, ejaculation, orgasm; impairments such as impotence, frigidity, vaginismus, premature ejaculation, priapism and delayed ejaculation

Exclusions: procreation functions (b660); sensations associated with genital and reproductive functions (b670)

      b 6400   **Functions of sexual arousal phase**
                 Functions of sexual interest and excitement.

      b 6401   **Functions of sexual preparatory phase**
                 Functions of engaging in sexual intercourse.

      b 6402   **Functions of orgasmic phase**
                 Functions of reaching orgasm.

      b 6403   **Functions of sexual resolution phase**
                 Functions of satisfaction after orgasm and accompanying relaxation.

Inclusions: impairments such as dissatisfaction with orgasm

b 6408   Sexual functions, other specified

b 6409   Sexual functions, unspecified

b 650   Menstruation functions
Functions associated with the menstrual cycle, including regularity of menstruation and discharge of menstrual fluids.

Inclusions: functions of regularity and interval of menstruation, extent of menstrual bleeding, menarche, menopause; impairments such as primary and secondary amenorrhoea, menorrhagia, polymenorrhoea and retrograde menstruation premenstrual tension

Exclusions: sexual functions (b640); procreation functions (b660); sensations associated with genital and reproductive functions (b670); sensation of pain (b280)

b 6500   Regularity of menstrual cycle
Functions involved in the regularity of the menstrual cycle.

Inclusions: too frequent or too few occurrences of menstruation

b 6501   Interval between menstruation
Functions relating to the length of time between two menstrual cycles.

b 6502   Extent of menstrual bleeding
Functions involved in the quantity of menstrual flow.

Inclusions: too little menstrual flow (hypomenorrhoea); too much menstrual flow (menorrhagia, hypermenorrhoea)

b 6503   Onset of menstruation
Functions related to the onset of the first menarche.

b 6508   Menstruation functions, other specified

b 6509   Menstruation functions, unspecified

b 660   Procreation functions
Functions associated with fertility, pregnancy, childbirth and lactation.

Inclusions: functions of male fertility and female fertility, pregnancy and childbirth, and lactation; impairments such as azoospermia, oligozoospermia, agalactorrhoea, galactorrhoea, alactationand such as in subfertility, sterility, spontaneous abortions, ectopic pregnancy, miscarriage, small fetus, hydramnios and premature childbirth, and delayed childbirth

Exclusions: sexual functions (b640); menstruation functions (b650)

b 6600 Functions related to fertility
Functions related to the ability to produce gametes for procreation.

Inclusion: impairments such as in subfertility and sterility

Exclusion: sexual functions (b640)

b 6601 Functions related to pregnancy
Functions involved in becoming pregnant and being pregnant.

b 6602 Functions related to childbirth
Functions involved during childbirth.

b 6603 Lactation
Functions involved in producing milk and making it available to the child.

b 6608 Procreation functions, other specified

b 6609 Procreation functions, unspecified

b 670 Sensations associated with genital and reproductive functions
Sensations arising from sexual arousal, intercourse, menstruation, and related genital or reproductive functions.

Inclusions: sensations of dyspareunia, dysmenorrhoea, hot flushes during menopause and night sweats during menopause

Exclusions: sensation of pain (b280); sensations associated with urinary functions (b630); sexual functions (b640); menstruation functions (b650); procreation functions (b660)

b 6700 Discomfort associated with sexual intercourse
Sensations associated with sexual arousal, preparation, intercourse, orgasm and resolution.

b 6701 Discomfort associated with the menstrual cycle
Sensations involved with menstruation, including pre-and post-menstrual phases.

b 6702 Discomfort associated with menopause
Sensations associated with cessation of the menstrual cycle.

Inclusions: hot flushes and night sweats during menopause

b 6703   Genital functions
Functions associated with arousal of the genitals.

Exclusions: sexual functions (b640); procreation functions (b660)

b 6708   Sensations associated with genital and reproductive functions, other specified

b 6709   Sensations associated with genital and reproductive functions, unspecified

b 679 Genital and reproductive functions, other specified and unspecified

b 698 Genitourinary and reproductive functions, other specified

b 699 Genitourinary and reproductive functions, unspecified

Chapter 7

Neuromusculoskeletal and movement-related functions

This chapter is about the functions of movement and mobility, including functions of joints, bones, reflexes and muscles.

Functions of the joints and bones (b710-b729)

b710   **Mobility of joint functions**
Functions of the range and ease of movement of a joint.

Inclusions: functions of mobility of single or several joints, vertebral, shoulder, elbow, wrist, hip, knee, ankle, small joints of hands and feet; mobility of joints generalized; impairments such as in hypermobility of joints, frozen joints, frozen shoulder, arthritis

Exclusions: stability of joint functions (b715); control of voluntary movement functions (b760)

     b 7100   **Mobility of a single joint**
                  Functions of the range and ease of movement of one joint.

     b 7101   **Mobility of several joints**
                  Functions of the range and ease of movement of more than one joint.

     b 7102   **Mobility of joints generalized**
                  Functions of the range and ease of movement of joints throughout the body.

     b 7108   **Mobility of joint functions, other specified**

     b 7109   **Mobility of joint functions, unspecified**

b715   **Stability of joint functions**
Functions of the maintenance of structural integrity of the joints.

Inclusions: functions of the stability of a single joint, several joints, and joints generalized; impairments such as in unstable shoulder joint, dislocation of a joint, dislocation of shoulder and hip

Exclusion: mobility of joint functions (b710)

     b 7150   **Stability of a single joint**
                  Functions of the maintenance of structural integrity of one joint.

b 7151   **Stability of several joints**
Functions of the maintenance of structural integrity of more than one joint.

b 7152   **Stability of joints generalized**
Functions of the maintenance of structural integrity of joints throughout the body.

b 7158   **Stability of joint functions, other specified**

b 7159   **Stability of joint functions, unspecified**

b 720 **Mobility of bone functions**
Functions of the range and ease of movement of the scapula, pelvis, carpal and tarsal bones.

Inclusions: impairments such as frozen scapula and frozen pelvis

Exclusion: mobility of joints functions (b710)

b 7200   **Mobility of scapula**
Functions of the range and ease of movement of the scapula.

Inclusions: impairments such as protraction, retraction, laterorotation and medial rotation of the scapula

b 7201   **Mobility of pelvis**
Functions of the range and ease of movement of the pelvis.

Inclusion: rotation of the pelvis

b 7202   **Mobility of carpal bones**
Functions of the range and ease of movement of the carpal bones.

b 7203   **Mobility of tarsal bones**
Functions of the range and ease of movement of the tarsal bones.

b 7208   **Mobility of bone functions, other specified**

b 7209   **Mobility of bone functions, specified**

b 729 **Functions of the joints and bones, other specified and unspecified**

Muscle functions (b730-b749)

b 730 **Muscle power functions**

Functions related to the force generated by the contraction of a muscle or muscle groups.

Inclusions: functions associated with the power of specific muscles and muscle groups, muscles of one limb, one side of the body, the lower half of the body, all limbs, the trunk and the body as a whole; impairments such as weakness of small muscles in feet and hands, muscle paresis, muscle paralysis, monoplegia, hemiplegia, paraplegia, quadriplegia and akinetic mutism

Exclusions: functions of structures adjoining the eye (b215); muscle tone functions (b735); muscle endurance functions (b740)

b 7300 **Power of isolated muscles and muscle groups**

Functions related to the force generated by the contraction of specific and isolated muscles and muscle groups.

Inclusions: impairments such as weakness of small muscles of feet or hands

b 7301 **Power of muscles of one limb**

Functions related to the force generated by the contraction of the muscles and muscle groups of one arm or leg.

Inclusions: impairments such as monoparesis and monoplegia

b 7302 **Power of muscles of one side of the body**

Functions related to the force generated by the contraction of the muscles and muscle groups found on the left or right side of the body.

Inclusions: impairments such as hemiparesis and hemiplegia

b 7303 **Power of muscles in lower half of the body**

Functions related to the force generated by the contraction of the muscles and muscle groups found in the lower half of the body.

Inclusions: impairments such as paraparesis and paraplegia

b 7304 **Power of muscles of all limbs**

Functions related to the force generated by the contraction of muscles and muscle groups of all four limbs.

Inclusions: impairments such as tetraparesis and tetraplegia

b 7305   Power of muscles of the trunk
Functions related to the force generated by the contraction of muscles and muscle groups in the trunk.

b 7306   Power of all muscles of the body
Functions related to the force generated by the contraction of all muscles and muscle groups of the body.

Inclusions: impairments such as akinetic mutism

b 7308   Muscle power functions, other specified

b 7309   Muscle power functions, unspecified

b 735   Muscle tone functions
Functions related to the tension present in the resting muscles and the resistance offered when trying to move the muscles passively.

Inclusions: functions associated with the tension of isolated muscles and muscle groups, muscles of one limb, one side of the body and the lower half of the body, muscles of all limbs, muscles of the trunk, and all muscles of the body; impairments such as hypotonia, hypertonia and muscle spasticity, myotonia and paramyotonia

Exclusions: muscle power functions (b730); muscle endurance functions (b740)

b 7350   Tone of isolated muscles and muscle groups
Functions related to the tension present in the resting isolated muscles and muscle groups and the resistance offered when trying to move those muscles passively.

Inclusions: impairments such as in focal dystonias, e.g. torticollis

b 7351   Tone of muscles of one limb
Functions related to the tension present in the resting muscles and muscle groups in one arm or leg and the resistance offered when trying to move those muscles passively.

Inclusions: impairments associated with monoparesis and monoplegia

b 7352   Tone of muscles of one side of body
Functions related to the tension present in the resting muscles and muscle groups of the right or left side of the body and the resistance offered when trying to move those muscles passively.

Inclusions: impairments associated with hemiparesis and hemiplegia

b 7353   Tone of muscles of lower half of body
Functions related to the tension present in the resting muscles and muscle groups in the lower half of the body and the resistance offered when trying to move those muscles passively.

Inclusions: impairments associated with paraparesis and paraplegia

b 7354   Tone of muscles of all limbs
Functions related to the tension present in the resting muscles and muscle groups in all four limbs and the resistance offered when trying to move those muscles passively.

Inclusions: impairments associated with tetraparesis and tetraplegia

b 7355   Tone of muscles of trunk
Functions related to the tension present in the resting muscles and muscle groups of the trunk and the resistance offered when trying to move those muscles passively.

b 7356   Tone of all muscles of the body
Functions related to the tension present in the resting muscles and muscle groups of the whole body and the resistance offered when trying to move those muscles passively.

Inclusions: impairments such as in generalized dystonias and Parkinson's disease, or general paresis and paralysis

b 7358   Muscle tone functions, other specified

b 7359   Muscle tone functions, unspecified

b 740   Muscle endurance functions
Functions related to sustaining muscle contraction for the required period of time.

Inclusions: functions associated with sustaining muscle contraction for isolated muscles and muscle groups, and all muscles of the body; impairments such as in myasthenia gravis

Exclusions: exercise tolerance functions (b455); muscle power functions (b730); muscle tone functions (b735)

b 7400   Endurance of isolated muscles
Functions related to sustaining muscle contraction of isolated muscles for the required period of time.

b 7401   **Endurance of muscle groups**
Functions related to sustaining muscle contraction of isolated muscle groups for the required period of time.

Inclusions: impairments associated with monoparesis, monoplegia, hemiparesis and hemiplegia, paraparesis and paraplegia

b 7402   **Endurance of all muscles of the body**
Functions related to sustaining muscle contraction of all muscles of the body for the required period of time.

Inclusions: impairments associated with tetraparesis, tetraplegia, general paresis and paralysis

b 7408   **Muscle endurance functions, other specified**

b 7409   **Muscle endurance functions, unspecified**

b 749   **Muscle functions, other specified and unspecified**

Movement functions (b750-b789)

b 750   **Motor reflex functions**
Functions of involuntary contraction of muscles automatically induced by specific stimuli.

Inclusions: functions of stretch motor reflex, automatic local joint reflex, reflexes generated by noxious stimuli and other exteroceptive stimuli; withdrawal reflex, biceps reflex, radius reflex, quadriceps reflex, patellar reflex, ankle reflex, appearance and persistence of reflexes

b 7500   **Stretch motor reflex**
Functions of involuntary contractions of muscles automatically induced by stretching.

b 7501   **Reflexes generated by noxious stimuli**
Functions of involuntary contractions of muscles automatically induced by painful or other noxious stimuli.

Inclusion: withdrawal reflex

b 7502   **Reflexes generated by other exteroceptive stimuli**
Functions of involuntary contractions of muscles automatically induced by external stimuli other than noxious stimuli.

Inclusion: rooting

b 7508   Motor reflex functions, other specified

b 7509   Motor reflex functions, unspecified

b 755   Involuntary movement reaction functions
Functions of involuntary contractions of large muscles or the whole body induced by body position, balance and threatening stimuli.

Inclusions: functions of postural reactions, righting reactions, body adjustment reactions, balance reactions, supporting reactions, defensive reactions

Exclusion: motor reflex functions (b750)

b 760   Control of voluntary movement functions
Functions associated with control over and coordination of voluntary movements.

Inclusions: functions of control of simple voluntary movements and of complex voluntary movements, coordination of voluntary movements, supportive functions of arm or leg, right left motor coordination, eye hand coordination, eye foot coordination; impairments such as control and coordination problems, e.g. clumsiness and dysdiadochokinesia

Exclusions: muscle power functions (b730); involuntary movement functions (b765); gait pattern functions (b770)

b 7600   Control of simple voluntary movements
Functions associated with control over and coordination of simple or isolated voluntary movements.

b 7601   Control of complex voluntary movements
Functions associated with control over and coordination of complex voluntary movements.

b 7602   Coordination of voluntary movements
Functions associated with coordination of simple and complex voluntary movements, performing movements in an orderly combination.

Inclusions: right left coordination, coordination of visually directed movements, such as eye hand coordination and eye foot coordination; impairments such as dysdiadochokinesia

b 7603   Supportive functions of arm or leg
Functions associated with control over and coordination of voluntary movements by placing weight either on the arms (elbows or hands) or on the legs (knees or feet).

b 7608   **Control of voluntary movement functions, other specified**

b 7609   **Control of voluntary movement functions, unspecified**

b 761 **Spontaneous movements**
Functions associated with frequency, fluency and complexity of total and individual body-part movements, such as infant spontaneous movements.

b 7610   **General movements**
Repertoire and quality of age-specific general spontaneous movements, such as "writhing" movements and "fidgety" movements in early life.

b 7611   **Specific spontaneous movements**
Repertoire and quality of other spontaneous movements normally present in the first postnatal months, such as arm and leg movements toward midline, finger movements and kicking.

b 7618   **Spontaneous movements, other specified**

b 7619   **Spontaneous movements, unspecified**

b 765 **Involuntary movement functions**
Functions of unintentional, non- or semi-purposive involuntary contractions of a muscle or group of muscles.

Inclusions: involuntary contractions of muscles; impairments such as tremors, tics, mannerisms, stereotypies, motor perseveration, chorea, athetosis, vocal tics, dystonic movements and dyskinesia

Exclusions: control of voluntary movement functions (b760); gait pattern functions (b770)

b 7650   **Involuntary contractions of muscles**
Functions of unintentional, non- or semi-purposive involuntary contractions of a muscle or group of muscles, such as those involved as part of a psychological dysfunction.

Inclusions: impairments such as choreatic and athetotic movements; sleep-related movement disorders

b 7651   **Tremor**
Functions of alternating contraction and relaxation of a group of muscles around a joint, resulting in shakiness.

b 7652 **Tics and mannerisms**
Functions of repetitive, quasi-purposive, involuntary contractions of a group of muscles.

Inclusion: impairments such as vocal tics, coprolalia and bruxism

b 7653 **Stereotypies and motor perseveration**
Functions of spontaneous, non-purposive movements such as repetitively rocking back and forth and nodding the head or wiggling.

b 7658 **Involuntary movement functions, other specified**

b 7659 **Involuntary movement functions, unspecified**

b 770 **Gait pattern functions**
Functions of movement patterns associated with walking, running or other whole body movements.

Inclusions: walking patterns and running patterns; impairments such as spastic gait, hemiplegic gait, paraplegic gait, asymmetric gait, limping and stiff gait pattern

Exclusions: muscle power functions (b730); muscle tone functions (b735); control of voluntary movement functions (b760); involuntary movement functions (b765)

b 780 **Sensations related to muscles and movement functions**
Sensations associated with the muscles or muscle groups of the body and their movement.

Inclusions: sensations of muscle stiffness and tightness of muscles, muscle spasm or constriction, and heaviness of muscles

Exclusion: sensation of pain (b280)

b 7800 **Sensation of muscle stiffness**
Sensation of tightness or stiffness of muscles.

b 7801 **Sensation of muscle spasm**
Sensation of involuntary contraction of a muscle or a group of muscles.

b 7808 **Sensations related to muscles and movement functions, other specified**

b 7809 **Sensations related to muscles and movement functions, unspecified**

b 789 **Movement functions, other specified and unspecified**

b 798   Neuromusculoskeletal and movement-related functions, other specified

b 799   Neuromusculoskeletal and movement-related functions, unspecified

Chapter 8

Functions of the skin and related structures

This chapter is about the functions of skin, nails and hair.

Functions of the skin (b810-b849)

b810 **Protective functions of the skin**
Functions of the skin for protecting the body from physical, chemical and biological threats.

Inclusions: functions of protecting against the sun and other radiation, photosensitivity, pigmentation, quality of skin; insulating function of skin, callus formation, hardening; impairments such as broken skin, ulcers, bedsores and thinning of skin

Exclusions: repair functions of the skin (b820); other functions of the skin (b830)

b820 **Repair functions of the skin**
Functions of the skin for repairing breaks and other damage to the skin.

Inclusions: functions of scab formation, healing, scarring; bruising and keloid formation

Exclusions: protective functions of the skin (b810); other functions of the skin (b830)

b830 **Other functions of the skin**
Functions of the skin other than protection and repair, such as cooling and sweat secretion.

Inclusions: functions of sweating, glandular functions of the skin and resulting body odour

Exclusions: protective functions of the skin (b810); repair functions of the skin (b820)

b840 **Sensation related to the skin**
Sensations related to the skin such as itching, burning sensation and tingling.

Inclusions: impairments such as pins and needles sensation and crawling sensation

Exclusion: sensation of pain (b280)

b849 **Functions of the skin, other specified and unspecified**

Functions of the hair and nails (b850-b869)

b 850   **Functions of hair**
Functions of the hair, such as protection, coloration and appearance.

Inclusions: functions of growth of hair, pigmentation of hair, location of hair; impairments such as loss of hair or alopecia

b 860   **Functions of nails**
Functions of the nails, such as protection, scratching and appearance.

Inclusions: growth and pigmentation of nails, quality of nails

b 869   **Functions of the hair and nails, other specified and unspecified**

b 898   **Functions of the skin and related structures, other specified**

b 899   **Functions of the skin and related structures, unspecified**

BODY STRUCTURES

Definitions: **Body structures** *are anatomical parts of the body such as organs, limbs and their components.*

Impairments *are problems in body function or structure as a significant deviation or loss.*

During childhood and adolescence, impairments may also take the form of delays or lags in the emergence of body structures in development.

First qualifier

Generic qualifier with the negative scale used to indicate the extent or magnitude of an impairment:

xxx.0	NO impairment	(none, absent, negligible,...)	0-4 %
xxx.1	MILD impairment	(slight, low,...)	5-24 %
xxx.2	MODERATE impairment	(medium, fair,...)	25-49 %
xxx.3	SEVERE impairment	(high, extreme, ...)	50-95 %
xxx.4	COMPLETE impairment	(total,...)	96-100 %
xxx.8	not specified		
xxx.9	not applicable		

Broad ranges of percentages are provided for those cases in which calibrated assessment instruments or other standards are available to quantify the impairment in body structure. For example, when "no impairment" or "complete impairment" in body structure is coded, this scaling may have margin of error of up to 5%. "Moderate impairment" is generally up to half of the scale of total impairment. The percentages are to be calibrated in different domains with reference to population standards as percentiles. For this quantification to be used in a uniform manner, assessment procedures need to be developed through research.

Second qualifier

Used to indicate the nature of the change in the respective body structure:

0 no change in structure
1 total absence
2 partial absence
3 additional part
4 aberrant dimensions
5 discontinuity
6 deviating position
7 qualitative changes in structure, including accumulation of fluid
8 not specified
9 not applicable

Third qualifier (suggested)

To be developed to indicate localization

0 more than one region
1 right
2 left
3 both sides
4 front
5 back
6 proximal
7 distal
8 not specified
9 not applicable

For a further explanation of coding conventions in ICF, refer to Annex 2.

Chapter 1

Structures of the nervous system

s 110   Structure of brain

  s 1100   Structure of cortical lobes

    s 11000   Frontal lobe

    s 11001   Temporal lobe

    s 11002   Parietal lobe

    s 11003   Occipital lobe

    s 11008   Structure of cortical lobes, other specified

    s 11009   Structure of cortical lobes, unspecified

  s 1101   Structure of midbrain

  s 1102   Structure of diencephalon

  s 1103   Basal ganglia and related structures

  s 1104   Structure of cerebellum

  s 1105   Structure of brain stem

    s 11050   Medulla oblongata

    s 11051   Pons

    s 11058   Structure of brain stem, other specified

    s 11059   Structure of brain stem, unspecified

  s 1106   Structure of cranial nerves

  s 1107   Structure of white matter

s 11070   Corpus callosum

s 11078   Structure of white matter, other specified

s 11079   Structure of white matter, unspecified

s 1108   Structure of brain, other specified

s 1109   Structure of brain, unspecified

s 120   Spinal cord and related structures

s 1200   Structure of spinal cord

s 12000   Cervical spinal cord

s 12001   Thoracic spinal cord

s 12002   Lumbosacral spinal cord

s 12003   Cauda equina

s 12008   Structure of spinal cord, other specified

s 12009   Structure of spinal cord, unspecified

s 1201   Spinal nerves

s 1208   Spinal cord and related structures, other specified

s 1209   Spinal cord and related structures, unspecified

s 130   Structure of meninges

s 140   Structure of sympathetic nervous system

s 150   Structure of parasympathetic nervous system

s 198   Structure of the nervous system, other specified

s 199   Structure of the nervous system, unspecified

Chapter 2

The eye, ear and related structures

s 210   Structure of eye socket

s 220   Structure of eyeball

        s 2200   Conjunctiva, sclera, choroid

        s 2201   Cornea

        s 2202   Iris

        s 2203   Retina

        s 2204   Lens of eyeball

        s 2205   Vitreous body

        s 2208   Structure of eyeball, other specified

        s 2209   Structure of eyeball, unspecified

s 230   Structures around eye

        s 2300   Lachrymal gland and related structures

        s 2301   Eyelid

        s 2302   Eyebrow

        s 2303   External ocular muscles

        s 2308   Structures around eye, other specified

        s 2309   Structures around eye, unspecified

s 240   Structure of external ear

s 250   Structure of middle ear

s 2500   Tympanic membrane

s 2501   Eustachian canal

s 2502   Ossicles

s 2508   Structure of middle ear, other specified

s 2509   Structure of middle ear, unspecified

s 260   Structure of inner ear

s 2600   Cochlea

s 2601   Vestibular labyrinth

s 2602   Semicircular canals

s 2603   Internal auditory meatus

s 2608   Structure of inner ear, other specified

s 2609   Structure of inner ear, unspecified

s 298   Eye, ear and related structures, other specified

s 299   Eye, ear and related structures, unspecified

Chapter 3

Structures involved in voice and speech

s 310   Structure of nose

> s 3100   External nose

> s 3101   Nasal septum

> s 3102   Nasal fossae

> s 3108   Structure of nose, other specified

> s 3109   Structure of nose, unspecified

s 320   Structure of mouth

> s 3200   Teeth

>> s 32000   Primary dentition

>> s 32001   Permanent dentition

>> s 32008   Teeth, other specified

>> s 32009   Teeth, unspecified

> s 3201   Gums

> s 3202   Structure of palate

>> s 32020   Hard palate

>> s 32021   Soft palate

> s 3203   Tongue

> s 3204   Structure of lips

>> s 32040   Upper lip

s 32041   Lower lip

s 3205   Philtrum

s 3208   Structure of mouth, other specified

s 3209   Structure of mouth, unspecified

s 330   Structure of pharynx

s 3300   Nasal pharynx

s 3301   Oral pharynx

s 3308   Structure of pharynx, other specified

s 3309   Structure of pharynx, unspecified

s 340   Structure of larynx

s 3400   Vocal folds

s 3408   Structure of larynx, other specified

s 3409   Structure of larynx, unspecified

s 398   Structures involved in voice and speech, other specified

s 399   Structures involved in voice and speech, unspecified

Chapter 4

Structures of the cardiovascular, immunological and respiratory systems

s 410   Structure of cardiovascular system

   s 4100   Heart

      s 41000   Atria

      s 41001   Ventricles

      s 41008   Structure of heart, other specified

      s 41009   Structure of heart, unspecified

   s 4101   Arteries

   s 4102   Veins

   s 4103   Capillaries

   s 4108   Structure of cardiovascular system, other specified

   s 4109   Structure of cardiovascular system, unspecified

s 420   Structure of immune system

   s 4200   Lymphatic vessels

   s 4201   Lymphatic nodes

   s 4202   Thymus

   s 4203   Spleen

   s 4204   Bone marrow

   s 4208   Structure of immune system, other specified

s 4209   Structure of immune system, unspecified

s 430   **Structure of respiratory system**

s 4300   Trachea

s 4301   Lungs

s 43010   Bronchial tree

s 43011   Alveoli

s 43018   Structure of lungs, other specified

s 43019   Structure of lungs, unspecified

s 4302   Thoracic cage

s 4303   Muscles of respiration

s 43030   Intercostal muscles

s 43031   Diaphragm

s 43038   Muscles of respiration, other specified

s 43039   Muscles of respiration, unspecified

s 4308   Structure of respiratory system, other specified

s 4309   Structure of respiratory system, unspecified

s 498   **Structures of the cardiovascular, immunological and respiratory systems, other specified**

s 499   **Structures of the cardiovascular, immunological and respiratory systems, unspecified**

Chapter 5

Structures related to the digestive, metabolic and endocrine systems

s 510   Structure of salivary glands

s 520   Structure of oesophagus

s 530   Structure of stomach

s 540   Structure of intestine

>   s 5400   Small intestine
>
>   s 5401   Large intestine
>
>   s 5408   Structure of intestine, other specified
>
>   s 5409   Structure of intestine, unspecified

s 550   Structure of pancreas

s 560   Structure of liver

s 570   Structure of gall bladder and ducts

s 580   Structure of endocrine glands

>   s 5800   Pituitary gland
>
>   s 5801   Thyroid gland
>
>   s 5802   Parathyroid gland
>
>   s 5803   Adrenal gland
>
>   s 5808   Structure of endocrine glands, other specified
>
>   s 5809   Structure of endocrine glands, unspecified

s 598   Structures related to the digestive, metabolic and endocrine systems, other specified

s 599   Structures related to the digestive, metabolic and endocrine systems, unspecified

Chapter 6

Structures related to the genitourinary and reproductive systems

s 610   Structure of urinary system

    s 6100   Kidneys

    s 6101   Ureters

    s 6102   Urinary bladder

    s 6103   Urethra

    s 6108   Structure of urinary system, other specified

    s 6109   Structure of urinary system, unspecified

s 620   Structure of pelvic floor

s 630   Structure of reproductive system

    s 6300   Ovaries

    s 6301   Structure of uterus

        s 63010   Body of uterus

        s 63011   Cervix

        s 63012   Fallopian tubes

        s 63018   Structure of uterus, other specified

        s 63019   Structure of uterus, unspecified

    s 6302   Breast and nipple

    s 6303   Structure of vagina and external genitalia

                       s 63030   Clitoris

                       s 63031   Labia majora

                       s 63032   Labia minora

                       s 63033   Vaginal canal

            s 6304   Testes and scrotum

            s 6305   Structure of the penis

                       s 63050   Glans penis

                       s 63051   Shaft of penis

                       s 63058   Structure of penis, other specified

                       s 63059   Structure of penis, unspecified

            s 6306   Prostate

            s 6308   Structures of reproductive system, other specified

            s 6309   Structures of reproductive system, unspecified

s 698   Structures related to the genitourinary and reproductive systems, other specified

s 699   Structures related to the genitourinary and reproductive systems, unspecified

Chapter 7

Structures related to movement

s 710   Structure of head and neck region

  s 7100   Bones of cranium

      s 71000   Sutures

      s 71001   Fontanelle

      s 71008   Bones of cranium, other specified

      s 71009   Bones of cranium, unspecified

  s 7101   Bones of face

  s 7102   Bones of neck region

  s 7103   Joints of head and neck region

  s 7104   Muscles of head and neck region

  s 7105   Ligaments and fasciae of head and neck region

  s 7108   Structure of head and neck region, other specified

  s 7109   Structure of head and neck region, unspecified

s 720   Structure of shoulder region

  s 7200   Bones of shoulder region

  s 7201   Joints of shoulder region

  s 7202   Muscles of shoulder region

  s 7203   Ligaments and fasciae of shoulder region

  s 7208   Structure of shoulder region, other specified

s 7209   Structure of shoulder region, unspecified

s 730   Structure of upper extremity

s 7300   Structure of upper arm

s 73000   Bones of upper arm

s 73001   Elbow joint

s 73002   Muscles of upper arm

s 73003   Ligaments and fasciae of upper arm

s 73008   Structure of upper arm, other specified

s 73009   Structure of upper arm, unspecified

s 7301   Structure of forearm

s 73010   Bones of forearm

s 73011   Wrist joint

s 73012   Muscles of forearm

s 73013   Ligaments and fasciae of forearm

s 73018   Structure of forearm, other specified

s 73019   Structure of forearm, unspecified

s 7302   Structure of hand

s 73020   Bones of hand

s 73021   Joints of hand and fingers

s 73022   Muscles of hand

s 73023   Ligaments and fasciae of hand

s 73028   Structure of hand, other specified

s 73029   Structure of hand, unspecified

s 7308   Structure of upper extremity, other specified

s 7309   Structure of upper extremity, unspecified

s 740   Structure of pelvic region

s 7400   Bones of pelvic region

s 7401   Joints of pelvic region

s 7402   Muscles of pelvic region

s 7403   Ligaments and fasciae of pelvic region

s 7408   Structure of pelvic region, other specified

s 7409   Structure of pelvic region, unspecified

s 750   Structure of lower extremity

s 7500   Structure of thigh

s 75000   Bones of thigh

s 75001   Hip joint

s 75002   Muscles of thigh

s 75003   Ligaments and fasciae of thigh

s 75008   Structure of thigh, other specified

s 75009   Structure of thigh, unspecified

s 7501   Structure of lower leg

s 75010   Bones of lower leg

s 75011   Knee joint

s 75012   Muscles of lower leg

s 75013   Ligaments and fasciae of lower leg

s 75018   Structure of lower leg, other specified

s 75019   Structure of lower leg, unspecified

s 7502   Structure of ankle and foot

s 75020   Bones of ankle and foot

s 75021   Ankle joint and joints of foot and toes

s 75022   Muscles of ankle and foot

s 75023   Ligaments and fasciae of ankle and foot

s 75028   Structure of ankle and foot, other specified

s 75029   Structure of ankle and foot, unspecified

s 7508   Structure of lower extremity, other specified

s 7509   Structure of lower extremity, unspecified

s 760   Structure of trunk

s 7600   Structure of vertebral column

s 76000   Cervical vertebral column

s 76001   Thoracic vertebral column

s 76002   Lumbar vertebral column

s 76003   Sacral vertebral column

s 76004   Coccyx

s 76008   Structure of vertebral column, other specified

s 76009   Structure of vertebral column, specified

s 7601   Muscles of trunk

s 7602   Ligaments and fasciae of trunk

s 7608   Structure of trunk, other specified

s 7609   Structure of trunk, unspecified

s 770   Additional musculoskeletal structures related to movement

s 7700   Bones

s 7701   Joints

s 7702   Muscles

s 7703   Extra-articular ligaments, fasciae, extramuscular aponeuroses, retinacula, septa, bursae, unspecified

s 7708   Additional musculoskeletal structures related to movement, other specified

s 7709   Additional musculoskeletal structures related to movement, unspecified

s 798   Structures related to movement, other specified

s 799   Structures related to movement, unspecified

Chapter 8

Skin and related structures

s 810 Structure of areas of skin

    s 8100   Skin of head and neck region

    s 8101   Skin of the shoulder region

    s 8102   Skin of upper extremity

    s 8103   Skin of pelvic region

    s 8104   Skin of lower extremity

    s 8105   Skin of trunk and back

    s 8108   Structure of areas of skin, other specified

    s 8109   Structure of areas of skin, unspecified

s 820 Structure of skin glands

    s 8200   Sweat glands

    s 8201   Sebaceous glands

    s 8208   Structure of skin glands, other specified

    s 8209   Structure of skin glands, unspecified

s 830 Structure of nails

    s 8300   Finger nails

    s 8301   Toe nails

    s 8308   Structure of nails, other specified

    s 8309   Structure of nails, unspecified

s 840   Structure of hair

      s 8400   Body hair

      s 8401   Facial hair

      s 8402   Axillary hair

      s 8403   Pubic hair

      s 8408   Structure of hair, other specified

      s 8409   Structure of hair, unspecified

s 898   Skin and related structures, other specified

s 899   Skin and related structures, unspecifed

ACTIVITIES AND PARTICIPATION

Definitions: **Activity** *is the execution of a task or action by an individual.*

Participation *is involvement in a life situation.*

Activity limitations *are difficulties an individual may have in executing activities.*

Participation restrictions *are problems an individual may experience in involvement in life situations.*

During childhood and adolescence, limitations and restrictions may also take the form of delays or lags in the emergence of activities and participation.

Qualifiers

The domains for the Activities and Participation component are given in a single list that covers the full range of life areas (from basic learning and watching to composite areas such as social tasks). This component can be used to denote activities (a) or participation (p) or both.

The two qualifiers for the Activities and Participation component are the *performance* qualifier and the *capacity* qualifier. The performance qualifier describes what an individual does in his or her current environment. Because the current environment brings in a societal context, performance as recorded by this qualifier can also be understood as "involvement in a life situation" or "the lived experience" of people in the actual context in which they live. This context includes the environmental factors – all aspects of the physical, social and attitudinal world, which can be coded using the Environmental Factors component.

The capacity qualifier describes an individual's ability to execute a task or an action. This qualifier identifies the highest probable level of functioning that a person may reach in a given domain at a given moment. Capacity is measured in a uniform or standard environment, and thus reflects the environmentally adjusted ability of the individual. The Environmental Factors component can be used to describe the features of this uniform or standard environment.

Both capacity and performance qualifiers can be used both with and without assistive devices or personal assistance, and in accordance with the following scale:

xxx.0	NO difficulty	(none, absent, negligible,…)	0-4 %
xxx.1	MILD difficulty	(slight, low,…)	5-24 %
xxx.2	MODERATE difficulty	(medium, fair,…)	25-49 %
xxx.3	SEVERE difficulty	(high, extreme, …)	50-95 %
xxx.4	COMPLETE difficulty	(total,…)	96-100 %
xxx.8	not specified		
xxx.9	not applicable		

Broad ranges of percentages are provided for those cases in which calibrated assessment instruments or other standards are available to quantify the performance problem or capacity limitation. For example, when no performance problem or a complete performance problem is coded, this scaling has a margin of error of up to 5%. A moderate performance problem is defined as up to half of the scale of a total performance problem. The percentages are to be calibrated in different domains with reference to population standards as percentiles. For this quantification to be used in a uniform manner, assessment procedures need to be developed through research.

For a further explanation of coding convention in ICF, refer to Annex 2.

Chapter 1

Learning and applying knowledge

This chapter is about learning, applying the knowledge that is learned, thinking, solving problems, and making decisions.

Purposeful sensory experiences (d110-d129)

d110　**Watching**
Using the sense of seeing intentionally to experience visual stimuli, such as visually tracking an object, watching persons, looking at a sporting event, person, or children playing.

d115　**Listening**
Using the sense of hearing intentionally to experience auditory stimuli, such as listening to a radio, the human voice, to music, a lecture, or to a story told.

d120　**Other purposeful sensing**
Using the body's other basic senses intentionally to experience stimuli, such as touching and feeling textures, tasting sweets or smelling flowers.

　　　d1200　**Mouthing**
　　　Exploring objects using mouth or lips.

　　　d1201　**Touching**
　　　Exploring objects using hands, fingers or other limbs or body parts.

　　　d1202　**Smelling**
　　　Exploring objects by bringing them to the nose or the nose to objects.

　　　d1203　**Tasting**
　　　Exploring the taste of food or liquid by biting, chewing, sucking.

d129　**Purposeful sensory experiences, other specified and unspecified**

Basic learning (d130-d159)

d130　**Copying**
Imitating or mimicking as a basic component of learning, such as copying, repeating a facial expression, a gesture, a sound or the letters of an alphabet.

Inclusion: immediate imitation of an action or behaviour

d 131 **Learning through actions with objects**
Learning through simple actions on a single object, two or more objects, symbolic and pretend play, such as in hitting an object, banging blocks and playing with dolls or cars.

> **d 1310** **Learning through simple actions with a single object**
> Simple actions on a single object or toy by manipulating, banging, moving, dropping, etc.

> **d 1311** **Learning through actions by relating two or more objects**
> Simple actions relating two or more objects, toys or other materials without regard for the specific features of the objects, toys or materials.

> **d 1312** **Learning through actions by relating two or more objects with regard to specific features**
> Actions relating two or more objects, toys or materials with regard to specific features, e.g. lid on box, cup on saucer.

> **d 1313** **Learning through symbolic play**
> Actions relating objects, toys or materials symbolically, such as feeding or dressing for a toy animal or doll.

> **d 1314** **Learning through pretend play**
> Actions involving pretence, substituting a novel object, body part or body movement to enact a situation or event, such as pretending that a block of wood is a car, pretending that a rolled up cloth is a doll.

> **d 1318** **Learning through actions, other specified**

> **d 1319** **Learning through actions, unspecified**

d 132 **Acquiring information**
Obtaining facts about persons, things and events, such as asking why, what, where and how, asking for names.

Exclusions: learning concepts (d137); acquiring skills (d155)

d 133 **Acquiring language**
Developing the competence to represent persons, objects, events and feelings through words, symbols, phrases and sentences.

Exclusions: acquiring additional language (d134); communication (d310-d399)

d 1330   Acquiring single words or meaningful symbols
Learning words or meaningful symbols, such as graphic or manual signs or symbols.

d 1331   Combining words into phrases
Learning to combine words into phrases.

d 1332   Acquiring syntax
Learning to produce appropriately constructed sentences or set of sentences.

d 1338   Acquiring language, other specified

d 1339   Acquiring language, unspecified

d 134   Acquiring additional language
Developing the competence to represent persons, objects, events, feelings through words, symbols, phrases and sentences, such as in an additional language or signing.

Exclusions: acquiring language (d133); communication (d310-d399)

d 135   Rehearsing
Repeating a sequence of events or symbols as a basic component of learning, such as counting by tens or practising the recitation of a rhyme with gestures, counting by tens or practising the recitation of a poem.

Inclusion: deferred imitation of an action or behaviour

d 137   Acquiring concepts
Developing competence to understand and use basic and complex concepts related to the characteristics of things, persons or events.

d 1370   Acquiring basic concepts
Learning to use such concepts as size, form, quantity, length, same, opposite.

d 1371   Acquiring complex concepts
Learning to use such concepts as classification, grouping, reversibility, seriation.

d 1378   Acquiring concepts, other specified

d 1379   Acquiring concepts, unspecified

d 140   Learning to read
Developing the competence to read written material (including Braille and other symbols) with fluency and accuracy, such as recognizing characters and alphabets, sounding out written words with correct pronunciation, and understanding words and phrases.

   d 1400   Acquiring skills to recognize symbols including figures, icons, characters, alphabet letters and words
   Learning elementary actions of deciphering letters and symbols, characters, and letters and words.

   d 1401   Acquiring skills to sound out written words
   Learning elementary actions of sounding out letters, symbols and words.

   d 1402   Acquiring skills to understand written words and phrases
   Learning elementary actions to grasp the meaning of written words and texts.

   d 1408   Learning to read, other specified

   d 1409   Learning to read, unspecified

d 145   Learning to write
Developing the competence to produce symbols that represent sounds, words or phrases in order to convey meaning (including Braille writing and other symbols), such as spelling effectively and using correct grammar.

   d 1450   Acquiring skills to use writing implements
   Learning elementary actions of writing down symbols or letters, such as holding a pencil, chalk or brush, writing a character or a symbol on a of piece paper, using a brailler, keyboard or peripheral device (mouse).

   d 1451   Acquiring skills to write symbols, characters and alphabet
   Learning elementary skills to transpose a sounded or a morpheme into a symbol or a character grapheme.

   d 1452   Acquiring skills to write words and phrases
   Learning elementary skills to transpose spoken words or ideas into written words or phrases.

   d 1458   Learning to write, other specified

   d 1459   Learning to write, unspecified

d 150   Learning to calculate
Developing the competence to manipulate numbers and perform simple and complex mathematical operations, such as using mathematical signs for addition and subtraction and applying the correct mathematical operation to a problem.

  d 1500   **Acquiring skills to recognize numerals, arithmetic signs and symbols**
  Learning elementary skills to recognize and use numbers, arithmetic signs and symbols.

  d 1501   **Acquiring skills of numeracy such as counting and ordering**
  Learning elementary skills to acquire the concept of numeracy and concepts of the sets.

  d 1502   **Acquiring skills in using basic operations**
  Learning arithmetic skills to use operations of addition, subtraction, multiplication.

  d 1508   **Learning to calculate, other specified**

  d 1509   **Learning to calculate, unspecified**

d 155   Acquiring skills
Developing basic and complex competencies in integrated sets of actions or tasks so as to initiate and follow through with the acquisition of a skill, such as manipulating tools or toys, or playing games.

Inclusions: acquiring basic and complex skills

Exclusions: learning to write (d145) and writing (d170), learning to play (d131)

  d 1550   **Acquiring basic skills**
  Learning elementary, purposeful actions, such as learning to wave in response, to use simple tools such as pencils and eating utensils.

  d 1551   **Acquiring complex skills**
  Learning integrated sets of actions so as to follow rules and to sequence and coordinate one's movements, such as learning to play games (e.g. football or chess) and to use a building tool.

  d 1558   **Acquiring skills, other specified**

  d 1559   **Acquiring skills, unspecified**

d 159   Basic learning, other specified and unspecified

Applying knowledge (d160-d179)

d 160 **Focusing attention**
Intentionally focusing on specific stimuli, such as by filtering out distracting noises.

> **d 1600** **Focusing attention on the human touch, face and voice**
> Intentionally attending to features of other persons, such as their face, touch or voice.

> **d 1601** **Focusing attention to changes in the environment**
> Intentionally attending to some element of the environment, such as changes in the quality, quantity or intensity of physical or social stimuli.

> **d 1608** **Focusing attention, other specified**

> **d 1609** **Focusing attention, unspecified**

d 161 **Directing attention**
Intentionally maintaining attention to specific actions or tasks for an appropriate length of time.

Exclusions: sustaining attention (b1400); undertaking a single task (d210); undertaking a complex task (d220)

d 163 **Thinking**
Formulating and manipulating ideas, concepts, and images, whether goal-oriented or not, either alone or with others, with types of thinking activities, such as pretending, playing with words, creating fiction, proving a theorem, playing with ideas, brainstorming, meditating, pondering, speculating or reflecting.

Exclusions: solving problems (d175); making decisions (d177)

> **d 1630** **Pretending**
> Engaging in make-believe activities involving imaginary persons, places, things or events.

> **d 1631** **Speculating**
> Manipulating ideas, concepts or images by guessing or assuming something based on incomplete facts or information.

> **d 1632** **Hypothesizing**
> Manipulating ideas, concepts or images involving the use of abstract thought to state assumptions or to test unproven facts.

> **d 1638** **Thinking, other specified**

d 1639   Thinking, unspecified

d 166   Reading
Performing activities involved in the comprehension and interpretation of written language (e.g. books, instructions, newspapers in text or Braille), for the purpose of obtaining general knowledge or specific information.

Inclusion: Comprehension and interpretation of written language in standard form of letters or characters as well as text created with unique symbols such as icons

Exclusion: learning to read (d140)

d 1660   Using general skills and strategies of the reading process
Recognizing words by applying phonetic and structural analysis and using contextual cues in reading aloud or in silence.

d 1661   Comprehending written language
Grasping the nature and meaning of written language in reading aloud or in silence.

d 1668   Reading, other specified

d 1669   Reading, unspecified

d 170   Writing
Using or producing symbols or language to convey information, such as producing a written record of events or ideas or drafting a letter.

Exclusion: learning to write (d145)

d 1700   Using general skills and strategies of the writing process
Applying words which convey appropriate meaning, employing conventional sentence structure.

d 1701   Using grammatical and mechanical conventions in written compositions
Applying standard spelling, punctuation and proper case forms, etc.

d 1702   Using general skills and strategies to complete compositions
Applying words and sentences to convey complex meaning and abstract ideas.

Exclusion: learning to write (d145)

d 1708   Writing, other specified

d1709 Writing, unspecified

d172 Calculating

Performing computations by applying mathematical principles to solve problems that are described in words and producing or displaying the results, such as computing the sum of three numbers or finding the result of dividing one number by another.

Exclusion: learning to calculate (d150)

d1720 Using simple skills and strategies of the calculation process
Applying concepts of numeracy, operations and sets to perform calculations.

d1721 Using complex skills and strategies of the calculation process
Applying mathematical procedures and methods such as algebra, calculus and geometry to solve problems.

d1728 Calculating, other specified

d1729 Calculating, unspecified

d175 Solving problems

Finding solutions to questions or situations by identifying and analysing issues, developing options and solutions, evaluating potential effects of solutions, and executing a chosen solution such as in resolving a dispute between two people.

Inclusions: solving simple and complex problems

Exclusions: thinking (d163); making decisions (d177)

d1750 Solving simple problems
Finding solutions to a simple problem involving a single issue or question, by identifying and analysing the issue, developing solutions, evaluating the potential effects of the solutions and executing a chosen solution.

d1751 Solving complex problems
Finding solutions to a complex problem involving multiple and interrelated issues, or several related problems, by identifying and analysing the issue, developing solutions, evaluating the potential effects of the solutions and executing a chosen solution.

d1758 Solving problems, other specified

d1759 Solving problems, unspecified

d 177   **Making decisions**
Making a choice among options, implementing the choice, and evaluating the effects of the choice, such as selecting and purchasing a specific item, or deciding to undertake and undertaking one task from among several tasks that need to be done.

Exclusions: thinking (d163); solving problems (d175)

d 179   **Applying knowledge, other specified and unspecified**

d 198   **Learning and applying knowledge, other specified**

d 199   **Learning and applying knowledge, unspecified**

Chapter 2

General tasks and demands

This chapter is about general aspects of carrying out single or multiple tasks, organizing routines and handling stress. These items can be used in conjunction with more specific tasks or actions to identify the underlying features of the execution of tasks under different circumstances.

d 210 **Undertaking a single task**
Carrying out simple or complex and coordinated actions related to the mental and physical components of a single task, such as initiating a task, organizing time, space and materials for a task, pacing task performance, and carrying out, completing and sustaining a task.

Inclusions: undertaking a simple or complex task; undertaking a single task independently or in a group

Exclusions: acquiring skills (d155); solving problems (d175); making decisions (d177); undertaking multiple tasks (d220)

> **d 2100** **Undertaking a simple task**
> Preparing, initiating and arranging the time and space required for a simple task; executing a simple task with a single major component, such as building a tower, putting on a shoe, reading a book, writing a letter, or making one's bed.

> **d 2101** **Undertaking a complex task**
> Preparing, initiating and arranging the time and space for a single complex task; executing a complex task with more than one component, which may be carried out in sequence or simultaneously, such as making up a place for playing, using several toys in make believe play, arranging the furniture in one's room or completing an assignment for school.

> **d 2102** **Undertaking a single task independently**
> Preparing, initiating and arranging the time and space for a simple or complex task; managing and executing a task on one's own and without the assistance of others, such as in solitary play involving sorting small objects, setting a table or building with blocks.

> **d 2103** **Undertaking a single task in a group**
> Preparing, initiating and arranging the time and space for a single task, simple or complex; managing and executing a task with people who are involved in some or all steps of the task, such as playing hide-and-seek, playing cards or board games with rules, or playing instruments together.

d 2104   Completing a simple task

Completing a simple task with a single major component, such as building a tower, putting on a shoe, reading a book, writing a letter, or making one's bed.

d 2105   Completing a complex task

Completing a complex task with more than one component, which may be carried out in sequence or simultaneously, such as making up a place for playing, using several toys in make believe play, arranging the furniture in one's room or completing an assignment for school.

d 2108   Undertaking single tasks, other specified

d 2109   Undertaking single tasks, unspecified

d 220   **Undertaking multiple tasks**

Carrying out simple or complex and coordinated actions as components of multiple, integrated and complex tasks in sequence or simultaneously.

Inclusions: undertaking multiple tasks; completing multiple tasks; undertaking multiple tasks independently and in a group

Exclusions: acquiring skills (d155); solving problems (d175); making decisions (d177); undertaking a single task (d210)

d 2200   Carrying out multiple tasks

Preparing, initiating and arranging the time and space needed for several tasks, and managing and executing several tasks, together or sequentially, such as dressing oneself completely for a cold day or making arrangements for a party.

d 2201   Completing multiple tasks

Completing several tasks, together or sequentially, such as getting up and getting ready to leave for school, shopping and completing errands for a friend while shopping.

d 2202   Undertaking multiple tasks independently

Preparing, initiating and arranging the time and space for multiple tasks, and managing and executing several tasks together or sequentially, on one's own and without the assistance of others.

d 2203   Undertaking multiple tasks in a group

Preparing, initiating and arranging the time and space for multiple tasks, and managing and executing several tasks together or sequentially with others who are involved in some or all steps of the multiple tasks.

d 2204 Completing multiple tasks independently
Completing multiple tasks independently, such as completing several assignments for homework, giving food and water to pets, setting the table and preparing dinner for the family.

d 2205 Completing multiple tasks in a group
Completing multiple tasks in a group, such as planning the time and place for a sporting event, inviting participants, securing the necessary sports equipment for participation and arranging transportation to and from the activity.

d 2208 Undertaking multiple tasks, other specified

d 2209 Undertaking multiple tasks, unspecified

d 230 Carrying out daily routine
Carrying out simple or complex and coordinated actions in order to plan, manage and complete the requirements of day-to-day procedures or duties, such as budgeting time and making plans for separate activities throughout the day.

Inclusions: managing and completing the daily routine; managing one's own activity level

Exclusion: undertaking multiple tasks (d220)

d 2300 Following routines
Responding to the guidance of others in engaging in basic daily procedures or duties.

d 2301 Managing daily routine
Carrying out simple or complex and coordinated actions in order to plan and manage the requirements of day-to-day procedures or duties.

d 2302 Completing the daily routine
Carrying out simple or complex and coordinated actions in order to complete the requirements of usual day-to-day procedures or duties, such as fulfilling the daily routines of awakening, getting dressed, eating breakfast, leaving for school or work and returning home at the end of the day.

d 2303 Managing one's own activity level
Carrying out actions and behaviours to arrange the requirements in energy and time day-to-day procedures or duties.

d 2304   Managing changes in daily routine
Making appropriate transitions in response to new requirements or changes in the usual sequence of activities such as finding another way to travel to school or work when public transport is unavailable.

d 2305   Managing one's time
Managing the time required to complete usual or specific activities, such as preparing to depart from the home, taking medications, and accessing assistive technology and supports.

d 2306   Adapting to time demands
Carrying out actions and behaviours appropriately in the required sequence and within the time allotted, such as running to the station when in danger of missing the train.

d 2308   Carrying out daily routine, other specified

d 2309   Carrying out daily routine, unspecified

d 240   Handling stress and other psychological demands
Carrying out simple or complex and coordinated actions to manage and control the psychological demands required to carry out tasks demanding significant responsibilities and involving stress, distraction, or crises, such as taking exams, driving a vehicle during heavy traffic, putting on clothes when hurried by parents, finishing a task within a time-limit or taking care of a large group of children.

Inclusions: handling responsibilities; handling stress and crisis

d 2400   Handling responsibilities
Carrying out simple or complex and coordinated actions to manage the duties of task performance and to assess the requirements of these duties.

d 2401   Handling stress
Carrying out simple or complex and coordinated actions to cope with pressure, emergencies or stress associated with task performance, such as waiting for one's turn, reciting in class, systematically looking for lost items and keeping track of time.

d 2402   Handling crisis
Carrying out simple or complex and coordinated actions to cope with decisive turning points in a situation or times of acute danger or difficulty, such as deciding the proper point at which to ask for help and to ask the right person for help.

d 2408   Handling stress and other psychological demands, other specified

d 2409   Handling stress and other psychological demands, unspecified

d 250   Managing one's own behaviour
Carrying out simple or complex and coordinated actions in a consistent manner in response to new situations, persons or experiences, such as being quiet in a library.

d 2500   Accepting novelty
Managing behaviour and expression of emotions in an appropriate accepting response to novel objects or situations.

d 2501   Responding to demands
Managing behaviour and expression of emotions in an appropriate manner in response to actual or perceived expectations or demands.

d 2502   Approaching persons or situations
Managing behaviour and expression of emotions in an appropriate pattern of initiating interactions with persons or in situations.

d 2503   Acting predictably
Managing behaviour and expression of emotions in a pattern of consistent effort in response to demands or expectations.

d 2504   Adapting activity level
Managing behaviour and expression of emotions with a pattern and level of energy appropriate to demands or expectations.

d 2508   Managing one's own behaviour, other specified

d 2509   Managing one's own behaviour, unspecified

d 298   General tasks and demands, other specified

d 299   General tasks and demands, unspecified

Chapter 3

Communication

This chapter is about general and specific features of communicating by language, signs and symbols, including receiving and producing messages, carrying on conversations, and using communication devices and techniques.

Communicating - receiving (d310-d329)

d310 **Communicating with - receiving - spoken messages**
Comprehending literal and implied meanings of messages in spoken language, such as understanding that a statement asserts a fact or is an idiomatic expression, such as responding and comprehending spoken messages.

  d 3100 **Responding to the human voice**
  Responding to the human voice in a very basic manner reflected by changes in breathing patterns, or with gross or fine body movements.

  d 3101 **Comprehending simple spoken messages**
  Responding appropriately in actions or with words to simple spoken messages (2-3 words) such as requests (e.g. give me) or commands (e.g. no, come here).

  d 3102 **Comprehending complex spoken messages**
  Responding appropriately in actions or with words to complex spoken messages (complete sentences), such as questions or instructions.

  d 3108 **Communicating with - receiving - spoken messages, other specified**

  d 3109 **Communicating with - receiving - spoken messages, unspecified**

d315 **Communicating with - receiving - nonverbal messages**
Comprehending the literal and implied meanings of messages conveyed by gestures, symbols and drawings, such as realizing that a child is tired when she rubs her eyes or that a warning bell means that there is a fire.

Inclusions: communicating with - receiving - body gestures, general signs and symbols, drawings and photographs

  d 3150 **Communicating with - receiving - body gestures**
  Comprehending the meaning conveyed by facial expressions, hand movements or signs, body postures, and other forms of body language.

d 3151   Communicating with - receiving - general signs and symbols
Comprehending the meaning represented by public signs and symbols, such as traffic signs, warning symbols, musical or scientific notations, and icons.

d 3152   Communicating with - receiving - drawings and photographs
Comprehending the meaning represented by drawings (e.g. line drawings, graphic designs, paintings, three-dimensional representations, pictograms), graphs, charts and photographs, such as understanding that an upward line on a height chart indicates that a child is growing.

d 3158   Communicating with - receiving - nonverbal messages, other specified

d 3159   Communicating with - receiving - nonverbal messages, unspecified

d 320   Communicating with - receiving - formal sign language messages
Receiving and comprehending messages in formal sign language with literal and implied meaning.

d 325   Communicating with - receiving - written messages
Comprehending the literal and implied meanings of messages that are conveyed through written language (including Braille), such as following political events in the daily newspaper or understanding the intent of religious scripture.

d 329   Communicating - receiving, other specified and unspecified

Communicating - producing (d330-d349)

d 330   Speaking
Producing words, phrases and longer passages in spoken messages with literal and implied meaning, such as expressing a fact or telling a story in oral language.

d 331   Pre-talking
Vocalizing when aware of another person in the proximal environment, such as producing sounds when the mother is close; babbling; babbling in turn-taking activities. Vocalizing in response to speech through imitating speech-sounds in a turn taking procedure.

d 332   Singing
Producing tones in a sequence resulting in a melody or performing songs on one's own or in a group.

d 335   Producing nonverbal messages
Using gestures, symbols and drawings to convey messages, such as shaking one's head to indicate disagreement or drawing a picture or diagram to convey a fact or complex idea.

Inclusions: producing body gestures, signs, symbols, drawings and photographs

d 3350   Producing body language
Conveying messages by intentional movements of the body, such as facial gestures (e.g. smiling, frowning, wincing), by arm and hand movements, and by postures (e.g. embracing to indicate affection or pointing to receive attention or an object).

d 3351   Producing signs and symbols
Conveying meaning by using signs and symbols (e.g. icons, Bliss board, scientific symbols) and symbolic notation systems, such as using musical notation to convey a melody.

d 3352   Producing drawings and photographs
Conveying meaning by drawing, painting, sketching, and making diagrams, pictures or photographs, such as drawing a map to give someone directions to a location.

d 3358   Producing nonverbal messages, other specified

d 3359   Producing nonverbal messages, unspecified

d 340   Producing messages in formal sign language
Conveying, with formal sign language, literal and implied meaning.

d 345   Writing messages
Producing the literal and implied meanings of messages that are conveyed through written language, such as writing a letter to a friend.

d 349   Communication - producing, other specified and unspecified

Conversation and use of communication devices and techniques (d350-d369)

d 350   Conversation
Starting, sustaining and ending an interchange of thoughts and ideas, carried out by means of spoken, written, sign or other forms of language, with one or more persons one knows or who are strangers, in formal or casual settings.

Inclusions: starting, sustaining and ending a conversation; conversing with one or many people

d 3500 Starting a conversation
Beginning an interchange, such as initiating turn-taking activity through eye-contact or other means, that leads to communication or dialogue, such as by introducing oneself, expressing customary greetings, or by introducing a topic or asking questions.

d 3501 Sustaining a conversation
Continuing an interchange by taking turns in vocalizing, speaking or using sign or shaping a dialogue by adding ideas, introducing a new topic or retrieving a topic that has been previously mentioned.

d 3502 Ending a conversation
Finishing an interchange or dialogue with customary termination statements or expressions and by bringing closure to the topic under discussion.

d 3503 Conversing with one person
Initiating, maintaining, shaping and terminating an interchange or dialogue with one person, such as in pre-verbal or verbal play, vocal or verbal exchange between mother and child, or in discussing the weather with a friend.

d 3504 Conversing with many people
Initiating, maintaining, shaping and terminating an interchange or dialogue with more than one individual, such as by starting and participating in a group interchange (e.g. in playing table games, in class discussion in school, or in informal or formal discussions).

d 3508 Conversation, other specified

d 3509 Conversation, unspecified

d 355 Discussion
Starting, sustaining and ending an examination of a matter, with arguments for or against, or debate carried out by means of spoken, written, sign or other forms of language, with one or more people one knows or who are strangers, in formal or casual settings.

Inclusion: discussion with one person or many people

d 3550 Discussion with one person
Initiating, maintaining, shaping or terminating an argument or debate with one person.

d 3551   Discussion with many people
Initiating, maintaining, shaping or terminating an argument or debate with more than one individual.

d 3558   Discussion, other specified

d 3559   Discussion, unspecified

d 360   Using communication devices and techniques
Using devices, techniques and other means for the purposes of communicating, such as calling a friend on the telephone.

Inclusions: using telecommunication devices, using writing machines and communication techniques

d 3600   Using telecommunication devices
Using telephones and other machines, such as facsimile or telex machines or computers (e-mail) as a means of communication.

d 3601   Using writing machines
Using machines for writing, such as typewriters, computers and Braille writers, as a means of communication.

d 3602   Using communication techniques
Performing actions and tasks involved in techniques for communicating, such as reading lips.

d 3608   Using communication devices and techniques, other specified

d 3609   Using communication devices and techniques, unspecified

d 369   Conversation and use of communication devices and techniques, other specified and unspecified

d 398   Communication, other specified

d 399   Communication, unspecified

Chapter 4

Mobility

This chapter is about moving by changing body position or location or by transferring from one place to another, by carrying, moving or manipulating objects, by walking, running or climbing, and by using various forms of transportation.

Changing and maintaining body position (d410-d429)

d 410 **Changing basic body position**
Getting into and out of a body position and moving from one location to another, such as rolling from one side to the other, sitting, standing, getting up out of a chair to lie down on a bed, and getting into and out of positions of kneeling or squatting.

Inclusion: changing body position from lying down, from squatting or kneeling, from sitting or standing, bending and shifting the body's centre of gravity

Exclusion: transferring oneself (d420)

d 4100 **Lying down**
Getting into and out of a lying down position or changing body position from horizonal to any other position, such as standing up or sitting down.

Inclusion: getting into a prostrate position

d 4101 **Squatting**
Getting into and out of the seated or crouched posture on one's haunches with knees closely drawn up or sitting on one's heels, such as may be necessary in toilets that are at floor level, or changing body position from squatting to any other position, such as standing up.

d 4102 **Kneeling**
Getting into and out of a position where the body is supported by the knees with legs bent, such as during prayers, or changing body position from kneeling to any other position, such as standing up.

d 4103 **Sitting**
Getting into and out of a seated position and changing body position from sitting down to any other position, such as standing up or lying down.

Inclusions: getting into a sitting position with bent legs or cross-legged; getting into a sitting position with feet supported or unsupported

d 4104   Standing
Getting into and out of a standing position or changing body position from standing to any other position, such as lying down or sitting down.

d 4105   Bending
Tilting the back downwards or to the side, at the torso, such as in bowing or reaching down for an object.

d 4106   Shifting the body's centre of gravity
Adjusting or moving the weight of the body from one position to another while sitting, standing or lying, such as moving from one foot to another while standing.

Exclusions: transferring oneself (d420); walking (d450)

d 4107   Rolling over
Moving the body from one position to another while lying, such as turning from side to side or from stomach to back.

d 4108   Changing basic body position, other specified

d 4109   Changing basic body position, unspecified

d 415   **Maintaining a body position**
Staying in the same body position as required, such as remaining seated or remaining standing for work or school.

Inclusions: maintaining a lying, squatting, kneeling, sitting and standing position

d 4150   Maintaining a lying position
Staying in a lying position for some time as required, such as remaining in a prone position in a bed.

Inclusions: staying in a prone (face down or prostrate), supine (face upwards) or side-lying position

d 4151   Maintaining a squatting position
Staying in a squatting position for some time as required, such as when sitting on the floor without a seat.

d 4152   Maintaining a kneeling position
Staying in a kneeling position where the body is supported by the knees with legs bent for some time as required, such as during prayers in church.

d 4153   Maintaining a sitting position
Staying in a seated position, on a seat or the floor, for some time as required, such as when sitting at a desk or table.

Inclusions: staying in a sitting position with straight legs or cross-legged, with feet supported or unsupported

d 4154   Maintaining a standing position
Staying in a standing position for some time as required, such as when standing in a queue.

Inclusions: staying in a standing position on a slope, on slippery or hard surfaces

d 4155   Maintaining head position
Controlling the position of the head and supporting its weight for a determined period of time.

d 4158   Maintaining a body position, other specified

d 4159   Maintaining a body position, unspecified

d 420   Transferring oneself
Moving from one surface to another, such as sliding along a bench or moving from a bed to a chair, without changing body position.

Inclusions: transferring oneself while sitting or lying

Exclusion: changing basic body position (d410)

d 4200   Transferring oneself while sitting
Moving from a sitting position on one seat to another seat on the same or a different level, such as moving from a chair to a bed.

Inclusions: moving from a chair to another seat, such as a toilet seat; moving from a wheelchair to a car seat

Exclusion: changing basic body position (d410)

d 4201   Transferring oneself while lying
Moving from one lying position to another on the same or a different level, such as moving from one bed to another.

Exclusion: changing basic body position (d410)

d 4208   **Transferring oneself, other specified**

d 4209   **Transferring oneself, unspecified**

d 429   **Changing and maintaining body position, other specified and unspecified**

Carrying, moving and handling objects (d430-d449)

d 430   **Lifting and carrying objects**
Raising up an object or taking something from one place to another, such as when lifting a cup or toy, or carrying a box or a child from one room to another.

Inclusions: lifting, carrying in the hands or arms, or on shoulders, hip, back or head; putting down

    d 4300   **Lifting**
    Raising up an object in order to move it from a lower to a higher level, such as when lifting a glass from the table.

    d 4301   **Carrying in the hands**
    Taking or transporting an object from one place to another using the hands, such as when carrying a drinking glass or a suitcase.

    d 4302   **Carrying in the arms**
    Taking or transporting an object from one place to another using the arms and hands, such as when carrying a pet or a child or other large object.

    d 4303   **Carrying on shoulders, hip and back**
    Taking or transporting an object from one place to another using the shoulders, hip or back, or some combination of these, such as when carrying a large parcel or school-bag.

    d 4304   **Carrying on the head**
    Taking or transporting an object from one place to another using the head, such when as carrying a container of water on the head.

    d 4305   **Putting down objects**
    Using hands, arms or other parts of the body to place an object down on a surface or place, such as when lowering a container of water to the ground.

    d 4308   **Lifting and carrying, other specified**

d 4309   Lifting and carrying, unspecified

d 435   Moving objects with lower extremities
Performing coordinated actions aimed at moving an object by using the legs and feet, such as kicking a ball or pushing pedals on a bicycle.

Inclusions: pushing with lower extremities; kicking

d 4350   Pushing with lower extremities
Using the legs and feet to exert a force on an object to move it away, such as pushing a chair away with a foot.

d 4351   Kicking
Using the legs and feet to propel something away, such as kicking a ball.

d 4358   Moving objects with lower extremities, other specified

d 4359   Moving objects with lower extremities, unspecified

d 440   Fine hand use
Performing the coordinated actions of handling objects, picking up, manipulating and releasing them using one's hand, fingers and thumb, such as required to lift coins off a table or turn a dial or knob.

Inclusions: picking up, grasping, manipulating and releasing

Exclusion: Lifting and carrying objects (d430)

d 4400   Picking up
Lifting or taking up a small object with hands and fingers, such as when picking up a pencil.

d 4401   Grasping
Using one or both hands to seize and hold something, such as when grasping a tool or a door knob.

d 4402   Manipulating
Using fingers and hands to exert control over, direct or guide something, such as when handling coins or other small objects, cutting with scissors, tying a shoelace, filling in colouring books, or using chopsticks or knife and fork.

d 4403   Releasing
Using fingers and hands to let go or set free something so that it falls or changes position, such as when dropping an item of clothing or a piece of food for a pet.

d 4408   Fine hand use, other specified

d 4409   Fine hand use, unspecified

d 445   Hand and arm use
Performing the coordinated actions required to move objects or to manipulate them by using hands and arms, such as when turning door handles or throwing or catching an object.

Inclusions: pulling or pushing objects; reaching; turning or twisting the hands or arms; throwing; catching

Exclusion: fine hand use (d440)

d 4450   Pulling
Using fingers, hands and arms to bring an object towards oneself or to move it from place to place, such as when pulling a string or closing a door.

d 4451   Pushing
Using fingers, hands and arms to move something from oneself or to move it from place to place, such as when pushing a toy or an animal away.

d 4452   Reaching
Using the hands and arms to extend outwards and touch and grasp something, such as when reaching across a table or desk for a book.

d 4453   Turning or twisting the hands or arms
Using fingers, hands and arms to rotate, turn or bend an object, such as is required to brush one's teeth or wash utensils.

d 4454   Throwing
Using fingers, hands and arms to lift something and propel it with some force through the air, such as when tossing a ball.

d 4455   Catching
Using fingers, hands and arms to grasp a moving object in order to bring it to a stop and hold it, such as when catching a ball.

d 4458   Hand and arm use, other specified

d 4459   Hand and arm use, unspecified

d 446 **Fine foot use**
Performing the coordinated actions to move or manipulate objects using one's foot and toes.

d 449 **Carrying, moving and handling objects, other specified and unspecified**

Walking and moving (d450–d469)

d 450 **Walking**
Moving along a surface on foot, step by step, so that one foot is always on the ground, such as when strolling, sauntering, walking forwards, backwards, or sideways.

Inclusions: walking short or long distances; walking on different surfaces; walking around obstacles

Exclusions: transferring oneself (d420); moving around (d455)

> **d 4500** **Walking short distances**
> Walking for less than a kilometre, such as walking around rooms or hallways, within a building or for short distances outside.

> **d 4501** **Walking long distances**
> Walking for more than a kilometre, such as across a village or town, between villages or across open areas.

> **d 4502** **Walking on different surfaces**
> Walking on sloping, uneven, or moving surfaces, such as on grass, gravel or ice and snow, or walking aboard a ship, train or other vehicle.

> **d 4503** **Walking around obstacles**
> Walking in ways required to avoid moving and immobile objects, people, animals, and vehicles, such as walking around a marketplace or shop, around or through traffic or other crowded areas.

> **d 4508** **Walking, other specified**

> **d 4509** **Walking, unspecified**

d 455 **Moving around**
Moving the whole body from one place to another by means other than walking, such as climbing over a rock or running down a street, skipping, scampering, jumping, somersaulting or running around obstacles.

Inclusions: crawling, climbing, running, jogging, jumping, swimming, scooting, rolling and shuffling

Exclusions: transferring oneself (d420); walking (d450)

d 4550   Crawling
Moving the whole body in a prone position from one place to another on hands, or hands and arms, and knees.

d 4551   Climbing
Moving the whole body upwards or downwards, over surfaces or objects, such as climbing steps, rocks, ladders or stairs, curbs or other objects.

d 4552   Running
Moving with quick steps so that both feet may be simultaneously off the ground.

d 4553   Jumping
Moving up off the ground by bending and extending the legs, such as jumping on one foot, hopping, skipping and jumping or diving into water.

d 4554   Swimming
Propelling the whole body through water by means of limb and body movements without taking support from the ground underneath.

d 4555   Scooting and rolling
Propelling the whole body from one place to another in a sitting or lying position without rising from the floor.

d 4556   Shuffling
Propelling the whole body from one place to another using legs but not lifting the feet off the floor or ground.

d 4558   Moving around, other specified

d 4559   Moving around, unspecified

d 460   Moving around in different locations
Walking and moving around in various places and situations, such as walking between rooms in a house, within a building, or down the street of a town.

Inclusions: moving around within the home, crawling or climbing within the home; walking or moving within buildings other than the home, and outside the home and other buildings

d 4600   Moving around within the home
Walking and moving around in one's home, within a room, between rooms, and around the whole residence or living area.

Inclusions: moving from floor to floor, on an attached balcony, courtyard, porch or garden

d 4601   Moving around within buildings other than home
Walking and moving around within buildings other than one's residence, such as moving around other people's homes, other private buildings, community and public buildings and enclosed areas.

Inclusions: moving throughout all parts of buildings and enclosed areas, between floors, inside, outside and around buildings, both public and private

d 4602   Moving around outside the home and other buildings
Walking and moving around close to or far from one's home and other buildings, without the use of transportation, public or private, such as walking for short or long distances around a town or village.

Inclusions: walking or moving down streets in the neighbourhood, town, village or city; moving between cities and further distances, without using transportation

d 4608   Moving around in different locations, other specified

d 4609   Moving around in different locations, unspecified

d 465   Moving around using equipment
Moving the whole body from place to place, on any surface or space, by using specific devices designed to facilitate moving or create other ways of moving around, such as with skates, skis, scuba equipment, swim fins, or moving down the street in a wheelchair or a walker.

Exclusions: transferring oneself (d420); walking (d450); moving around (d455); using transportation (d470); driving (d475)

d 469   Walking and moving, other specified and unspecified

Moving around using transportation (d470–d489)

d 470   Using transportation
Using transportation to move around as a passenger, such as being driven in a car, bus, rickshaw, jitney, pram or stroller, animal-powered vehicle, private or public taxi, train, tram, subway, boat or aircraft.

Inclusions: using human-powered transportation; using private motorized or public transportation

Exclusions: moving around using equipment (d465); driving (d475)

d 4700   Using human-powered vehicles
Being transported as a passenger by a mode of transportation powered by one or more people, such as riding in a pram, stroller, rickshaw or rowboat.

d 4701   Using private motorized transportation
Being transported as a passenger by private motorized vehicle over land, sea or air, such as by car, taxi or privately-owned aircraft or boat.

d 4702   Using public motorized transportation
Being transported as a passenger by a motorized vehicle over land, sea or air designed for public transportation, such as being a passenger on a bus, train, subway or aircraft.

d 4703   Using humans for transportation
Being transported by another person, such as in a sheet, a backpack or a transportation device.

d 4708   Using transportation, other specified

d 4709   Using transportation, unspecified

d 475   Driving
Being in control of and moving a vehicle or the animal that draws it, travelling under one's own direction or having at one's disposal any form of transportation, such as a car, bicycle, boat or animal-powered vehicle.

Inclusions: driving human-powered transportation, motorized vehicles, animal-powered vehicles

Exclusions: moving around using equipment (d465); using transportation (d470)

d 4750   Driving human-powered transportation
Driving a human-powered vehicle, such as a bicycle, tricycle, or rowboat.

d 4751   Driving motorized vehicles
Driving a vehicle with a motor, such as an automobile, motorcycle, motorboat or aircraft.

d 4752 **Driving animal-powered vehicles**
Driving a vehicle powered by an animal, such as a horse-drawn cart or carriage.

d 4758 **Driving, other specified**

d 4759 **Driving, unspecified**

d 480 **Riding animals for transportation**
Travelling on the back of an animal, such as a horse, ox, camel or elephant.

Exclusions: driving (d475); recreation and leisure (d920)

d 489 **Moving around using transportation, other specified and unspecified**

d 498 **Mobility, other specified**

d 499 **Mobility, unspecified**

Chapter 5

Self-care

This chapter is about caring for oneself, washing and drying oneself, caring for one's body and body parts, dressing, eating and drinking, and looking after one's health.

d510 **Washing oneself**
Washing and drying one's whole body, or body parts, using water and appropriate cleaning and drying materials or methods, such as bathing, showering, washing hands and feet, face and hair, and drying with a towel.

Inclusions: washing body parts, the whole body; and drying oneself

Exclusions: caring for body parts (d520); toileting (d530)

> **d 5100** **Washing body parts**
> Applying water, soap and other substances to body parts, such as hands, face, feet, hair or nails, in order to clean them.

> **d 5101** **Washing whole body**
> Applying water, soap and other substances to the whole body in order to clean oneself, such as taking a bath or shower.

> **d 5102** **Drying oneself**
> Using a towel or other means for drying some part or parts of one's body, or the whole body, such as after washing.

> **d 5108** **Washing oneself, other specified**

> **d 5109** **Washing oneself, unspecified**

d520 **Caring for body parts**
Looking after those parts of the body, such as skin, face, teeth, scalp, nails and genitals, that require more than washing and drying.

Inclusions: caring for skin, teeth, hair, finger and toe nails, and nose

Exclusions: washing oneself (d510); toileting (d530)

> **d 5200** **Caring for skin**
> Looking after the texture and hydration of one's skin, such as by removing calluses or corns and using moisturizing lotions or cosmetics.

d 5201   Caring for teeth
Looking after dental hygiene, such as by brushing teeth, flossing, and taking care of a dental prosthesis or orthosis.

d 5202   Caring for hair
Looking after the hair on the head and face, such as by combing, styling, shaving, or trimming.

d 5203   Caring for fingernails
Cleaning, trimming or polishing the nails of the fingers.

d 5204   Caring for toenails
Cleaning, trimming or polishing the nails of the toes.

d 5205   Caring for nose
Cleaning the nose, looking after nasal hygiene.

d 5208   Caring for body parts, other specified

d 5209   Caring for body parts, unspecified

d 530   Toileting
Indicating the need for, planning and carrying out the elimination of human waste (menstruation, urination and defecation), and cleaning oneself afterwards.

Inclusions: regulating urination, defecation and menstrual care

Exclusions: washing oneself (d510); caring for body parts (d520)

d 5300   Regulating urination
Coordinating and managing urination, such as by indicating need, getting into the proper position, choosing and getting to an appropriate place for urination, manipulating clothing before and after urination, and cleaning oneself after urination.

d 53000   Indicating need for urination

d 53001   Carrying out urination appropriately

d 53008   Regulating urination, other specified

d 53009   Regulating urination, unspecified

d 5301   Regulating defecation
Coordinating and managing defecation such as by indicating need, getting into the proper position, choosing and getting to an appropriate place for defecation, manipulating clothing before and after defecation, and cleaning oneself after defecation.

> **d 53010   Indicating need for defecation**

> **d 53011   Carrying out defecation appropriately**

> **d 53018   Regulating defecation, other specified**

> **d 53019   Regulating defecation, unspecified**

d 5302   Menstrual care
Coordinating, planning and caring for menstruation, such as by anticipating menstruation and using sanitary towels and napkins.

d 5308   Toileting, other specified

d 5309   Toileting, unspecified

d 540   Dressing

Carrying out the coordinated actions and tasks of putting on and taking off clothes and footwear in sequence and in keeping with climatic and social conditions, such as by putting on, adjusting and removing shirts, skirts, blouses, pants, undergarments, saris, kimono, tights, hats, gloves, coats, shoes, boots, sandals and slippers.

Inclusions: putting on or taking off clothes and footwear and choosing appropriate clothing

d 5400   Putting on clothes
Carrying out the coordinated tasks of putting clothes on various parts of the body, such as putting clothes on over the head, over the arms and shoulders, and on the lower and upper halves of the body; putting on gloves and headgear.

d 5401   Taking off clothes
Carrying out the coordinated tasks of taking clothes off various parts of the body, such as pulling clothes off and over the head, off the arms and shoulders, and off the lower and upper halves of the body; taking off gloves and headgear.

d 5402 Putting on footwear
Carrying out the coordinated tasks of putting on socks, stockings and footwear.

d 5403 Taking off footwear
Carrying out the coordinated tasks of taking off socks, stockings and footwear.

d 5404 Choosing appropriate clothing
Following implicit or explicit dress codes and conventions of one's society or culture and dressing in keeping with climatic conditions.

d 5408 Dressing, other specified

d 5409 Dressing, unspecified

d 550 Eating
Indicating need for, and carrying out the coordinated tasks and actions of eating food that has been served, bringing it to the mouth and consuming it in culturally acceptable ways, cutting or breaking food into pieces, opening bottles and cans, using eating implements, having meals, feasting or dining.

Exclusion: drinking (d560)

d 5500 Indicating need for eating

d 5501 Carrying out eating appropriately

d 5508 Eating, other specified

d 5509 Eating, unspecified

d 560 Drinking
Indicating need for, and taking hold of a drink, bringing it to the mouth and consuming the drink in culturally acceptable ways; mixing, stirring and pouring liquids for drinking, opening bottles and cans, drinking through a straw or drinking running water, such as from a tap or a spring; feeding from the breast.

Exclusion: eating (d550)

d 5600 Indicating need for drinking

d 5601   Carrying out breast feeding

Successfully suckle breast for milk and appropriate behaviours and interactions with caregiver, such as eye contact, indicating need and satiation.

d 5602   Carrying out feeding from bottle

Successfully suckle from a bottle for milk or other liquid and appropriate behaviours and interactions with caregiver, such as eye contact, indicating need and satiation.

d 5608   Drinking, other specified

d 5609   Drinking, unspecified

d 570   Looking after one's health

Ensuring or indicating needs about physical comfort, health and physical and mental well-being, such as by maintaining a balanced diet and an appropriate level of physical activity, keeping warm or cool, avoiding harm to health, following safe sex practices, including using condoms, getting immunizations and regular physical examinations.

Inclusions: ensuring one's physical comfort; managing diet and fitness; maintaining one's health

d 5700   Ensuring one's physical comfort

Caring for oneself by being aware that one needs to ensure, and ensuring, that one's body is in a comfortable position, that one is not feeling too hot, cold or wet, and that one has adequate lighting.

d 5701   Managing diet and fitness

Caring for oneself by being aware of the need and by selecting and consuming nutritious foods and maintaining physical fitness.

d 5702   Maintaining one's health

Caring for oneself by being aware of the need and doing what is required to look after one's health, both to respond to risks to health and to prevent ill-health, such as by seeking caregiver or professional assistance; following medical and other health advice; and avoiding risks to health such as physical injury, communicable diseases, drug-taking and sexually transmitted diseases.

d 57020   Managing medications and following health advice

d 57021   Seeking advice or assistance from caregivers or professionals

          d 57022   Avoiding risks of abuse of drugs or alcohol

          d 57028   Maintaining one's health, other specified

          d 57029   Maintaining one's health, unspecified

     d 5708   Looking after one's health, other specified

     d 5709   Looking after one's health, unspecified

d 571   **Looking after one's safety**
Avoiding risks that can lead to physical injury or harm. Avoiding potentially hazardous situations such as misusing fire or running into traffic.

d 598   **Self-care, other specified**

d 599   **Self-care, unspecified**

Chapter 6

Domestic life

This chapter is about carrying out domestic and everyday actions and tasks. Areas of domestic life include acquiring a place to live, food, clothing and other necessities, household cleaning and repairing, caring for personal and other household objects, and assisting others.

Acquisition of necessities (d610-d629)

d610 **Acquiring a place to live**
Buying, renting, furnishing and arranging a room, house, apartment or other dwelling.

Inclusions: buying or renting a place to live and furnishing a place to live

Exclusions: acquisition of goods and services (d620); caring for household objects (d650)

d 6100 **Buying a place to live**
Acquiring ownership of a house, apartment or other dwelling.

d 6101 **Renting a place to live**
Acquiring the use of a house, apartment or other dwelling belonging to another in exchange for payment.

d 6102 **Furnishing a place to live**
Equipping and arranging a living space with furniture, fixtures and other fittings and decorating rooms, arranging one's own space, room.

d 6108 **Acquiring a place to live, other specified**

d 6109 **Acquiring a place to live, unspecified**

d620 **Acquisition of goods and services**
Selecting, procuring and transporting all goods and services required for daily living, such as selecting, procuring, transporting and storing food, drink, clothing, cleaning materials, fuel, household items, utensils, cooking ware, play-material, domestic appliance and tools; procuring utilities and other household services.

Inclusions: shopping and gathering daily necessities

Exclusion: acquiring a place to live (d610)

d 6200   Shopping
Obtaining, in exchange for money, goods and services required for daily living (including instructing and supervising an intermediary to do the shopping), such as selecting food, drink, cleaning materials, household items, play-material or clothing in a shop or market; comparing quality and price of the items required, negotiating and paying for selected goods or services, and transporting goods.

d 6201   Gathering daily necessities
Obtaining, without exchange of money, goods and services required for daily living (including instructing and supervising an intermediate to gather daily necessities), such as by harvesting vegetables and fruits and getting water and fuel.

d 6208   Acquisition of goods and services, other specified

d 6209   Acquisition of goods and services, unspecified

d 629   Acquisition of necessities, other specified and unspecified

Household tasks (d630-d649)

d 630   Preparing meals
Planning, organizing, cooking and serving simple and complex meals for oneself and others, such as by making a menu, selecting edible food and drink, getting together ingredients for preparing meals, cooking with heat and preparing cold foods and drinks, and serving the food.

Inclusions: preparing simple and complex meals

Exclusions: eating (d550); drinking (d560); acquisition of goods and services (d620); doing housework (d640); caring for household objects (d650); caring for others (d660)

d 6300   Preparing simple meals
Organizing, cooking and serving meals with a small number of ingredients that require easy methods of preparation and serving, such as making a snack or small meal, and transforming food ingredients by cutting and stirring, boiling and heating food such as rice or potatoes.

d 6301   Preparing complex meals
Planning, organizing, cooking and serving meals with a large number of ingredients that require complex methods of preparation and serving, such as planning a meal with several dishes, and transforming food

ingredients by combined actions of peeling, slicing, mixing, kneading, stirring, presenting and serving food in a manner appropriate to the occasion and culture.

Exclusion: using household appliances (d6403)

d 6302   Helping prepare meals
Working with others in planning, organizing, cooking and serving simple and complex meals for oneself and others, with someone else in charge.

d 6308   Preparing meals, other specified

d 6309   Preparing meals, unspecified

d 640   Doing housework
Managing a household by cleaning the house, washing clothes, using household appliances, storing food and disposing of garbage, such as by sweeping, mopping, washing counters, walls and other surfaces; collecting and disposing of household garbage; tidying rooms, closets and drawers; collecting, washing, drying, folding and ironing clothes; cleaning footwear; using brooms, brushes and vacuum cleaners; using washing machines, driers and irons.

Inclusions: washing and drying clothes and garments; cleaning cooking area and utensils; cleaning living area; using household appliances, storing daily necessities and disposing of garbage

Exclusions: acquiring a place to live (d610); acquisition of goods and services (d620); preparing meals (d630); caring for household objects (d650); caring for others (d660)

d 6400   Washing and drying clothes and garments
Washing clothes and garments by hand and hanging them out to dry in the air.

d 6401   Cleaning cooking area and utensils
Cleaning up after cooking, such as by washing dishes, pans, pots and cooking utensils, and cleaning tables and floors around cooking and eating area.

d 6402   Cleaning living area
Cleaning the living areas of the household, such as by tidying and dusting, sweeping, swabbing, mopping floors, cleaning windows and walls, cleaning bathrooms and toilets, cleaning household furnishings.

d 6403   Using household appliances
Using all kinds of household appliances, such as washing machines, driers, irons, vacuum cleaners and dishwashers.

d 6404 **Storing daily necessities**
Storing food, drinks, clothes and other household goods required for daily living; preparing food for conservation by canning, salting or refrigerating, keeping food fresh and out of the reach of animals.

d 6405 **Disposing of garbage**
Disposing of household garbage such as by collecting trash and rubbish around the house, preparing garbage for disposal, using garbage disposal appliances; burning garbage.

d 6406 **Helping to do housework**
Working with others in planning, organizing and managing a household, with someone else in charge.

d 6408 **Doing housework, other specified**

d 6409 **Doing housework, unspecified**

d 649 Household tasks, other specified and unspecified

Caring for household objects and assisting others (d650-d669)

d 650 Caring for household objects
Maintaining and repairing household and other personal objects, including play-material, house and contents, clothes, vehicles and assistive devices, and caring for plants and animals, such as painting or wallpapering rooms, fixing furniture, repairing plumbing, ensuring the proper working order of vehicles, watering plants, grooming and feeding pets and domestic animals.

Inclusions: making and repairing clothes; maintaining dwelling, furnishings and domestic appliances; maintaining vehicles; maintaining assistive devices; taking care of plants (indoor and outdoor) and animals

Exclusions: acquiring a place to live (d610); acquisition of goods and services (d620); doing housework (d640); caring for others (d660); remunerative employment (d850)

d 6500 **Making and repairing clothes**
Making and repairing clothes, such as by sewing, producing or mending clothes; reattaching buttons and fasteners; ironing clothes, fixing and polishing footwear.

Exclusion: using household appliances (d6403)

d 6501 **Maintaining dwelling and furnishings**
Repairing and taking care of dwelling, its exterior, interior and contents,

such as by painting, repairing fixtures and furniture, and using required tools for repair work.

d 6502   Maintaining domestic appliances
Repairing and taking care of all domestic appliances for cooking, cleaning and repairing, such as by oiling and repairing tools and maintaining the washing machine.

d 6503   Maintaining vehicles
Repairing and taking care of motorized and non-motorized vehicles for personal use, including bicycles, carts, automobiles and boats.

d 6504   Maintaining assistive devices
Repairing and taking care of assistive devices, such as prostheses, orthoses and specialized tools and aids for housekeeping and personal care; maintaining and repairing aids for personal mobility such as canes, walkers, wheelchairs and scooters; and maintaining communication and recreational aids.

d 6505   Taking care of plants, indoors and outdoors
Taking care of plants inside and outside the house, such as by planting, watering and fertilizing plants; gardening and growing foods for personal use.

d 6506   Taking care of animals
Taking care of domestic animals and pets, such as by feeding, cleaning, grooming and exercising pets; watching over the health of animals or pets; planning for the care of animals or pets in one's absence.

d 6507   Helping to care for household objects
Working with others in maintaining and repairing household and other personal objects, with someone else in charge.

d 6508   Caring for household objects, other specified

d 6509   Caring for household objects, unspecified

d 660   Assisting others
Assisting household members and others with their learning, communicating, self-care, movement, within the house or outside; being concerned about, or drawing other's attention to, the well-being of household members and others.

Inclusions: assisting others with self-care, movement, communication, interpersonal relations, nutrition and health maintenance

Exclusion: remunerative employment (d850)

d 6600   Assisting others with self-care
Assisting household members and others in performing self-care, including helping others with eating, bathing and dressing; taking care of children or members of the household who are sick or have difficulties with basic self-care; helping others with their toileting.

d 6601   Assisting others in movement
Assisting household members and others in movements and in moving outside the home, such as in the neighbourhood or city, to or from school, place of employment or other destination.

d 6602   Assisting others in communication
Assisting household members and others with their communication, such as by helping with speaking, writing or reading.

d 6603   Assisting others in interpersonal relations
Assisting household members and others with their interpersonal interactions, such as by helping them to initiate, maintain or terminate relationships.

d 6604   Assisting others in nutrition
Assisting household members and others with their nutrition, such as by helping them to prepare and eat meals.

d 6605   Assisting others in health maintenance
Assisting household members and others with formal and informal health care, such as by ensuring that a child gets regular medical check-ups, or that an elderly relative takes required medication.

d 6606   Helping in assisting others
Helping in the provision of assistance to household members and others with self-care, communication, movement, interpersonal relations, nutrition and health maintenance, with someone else in charge.

d 6608   Assisting others, other specified

d 6609   Assisting others, unspecified

d 669   Caring for household objects and assisting others, other specified and unspecified

d 698   Domestic life, other specified

d 699   Domestic life, unspecified

Chapter 7

Interpersonal interactions and relationships

This chapter is about carrying out the actions and tasks required for basic and complex interactions with people (strangers, friends, relatives, family members and lovers) in a contextually and socially appropriate manner.

General interpersonal interactions (d710-d729)

d710 **Basic interpersonal interactions**
Interacting with people in a contextually and socially appropriate manner, such as by showing consideration and esteem when appropriate, or responding to the feelings of others.

Inclusions: showing respect, warmth, appreciation, and tolerance in relationships; responding to criticism and social cues in relationships; and using appropriate physical contact in relationships

> **d7100** **Respect and warmth in relationships**
> Showing and responding to concerns, sympathy, consideration and esteem in a contextually and socially appropriate manner.

> **d7101** **Appreciation in relationships**
> Showing and responding to satisfaction and gratitude in a contextually and socially appropriate manner.

> **d7102** **Tolerance in relationships**
> Showing and responding to understanding and acceptance of behaviour in a contextually and socially appropriate manner.

> **d7103** **Criticism in relationships**
> Providing and responding to implicit and explicit differences of opinion or disagreement in a contextually and socially appropriate manner.

> **d7104** **Social cues in relationships**
> Giving and reacting appropriately to signs and hints that occur in social interactions.

>> **d71040** **Initiating social interactions**
>> Initiating and responding appropriately in reciprocal social exchange with others.

>> **d71041** **Maintaining social interactions**
>> Regulating behaviours to sustain social exchanges.

d 71048   Social cues in relationships, other specified

d 71049   Social cues in relationships, unspecified

d 7105   Physical contact in relationships
Making and responding to bodily contact with others, in a contextually and socially appropriate manner.

d 7106   Differentiation of familiar persons
Showing differential responses to individuals, such as by reaching out for the familiar person and differentiating them from strangers.

d 7108   Basic interpersonal interactions, other specified

d 7109   Basic interpersonal interactions, unspecified

d 720   Complex interpersonal interactions
Maintaining and managing interactions with other people, in a contextually and socially appropriate manner, such as by regulating emotions and impulses, controlling verbal and physical aggression, acting independently in social interactions, and acting in accordance with social rules and conventions.

Inclusions: playing with others, forming and terminating relationships; regulating behaviours within interactions; interacting according to social rules; and maintaining social space

d 7200   Forming relationships
Beginning and maintaining interactions with others for a short or long period of time, in a contextually and socially appropriate manner, such as by introducing oneself, finding and establishing friendships and professional relationships, starting a relationship that may become permanent, romantic or intimate.

d 7201   Terminating relationships
Bringing interactions to a close in a contextually and socially appropriate manner, such as by ending temporary relationships at the end of a visit, ending long-term relationships with friends when moving to a new town or ending relationships with work colleagues, professional colleagues and service providers, and ending romantic or intimate relationships.

d 7202   Regulating behaviours within interactions
Regulating emotions and impulses, verbal aggression and physical aggression in interactions with others, in a contextually and socially appropriate manner.

> **d 7203   Interacting according to social rules**
> Acting independently in social interactions and complying with social conventions governing one's role, position or other social status in interactions with others.

> **d 7204   Maintaining social space**
> Being aware of and maintaining a distance between oneself and others that is contextually, socially and culturally appropriate.

> **d 7208   Complex interpersonal interactions, other specified**

> **d 7209   Complex interpersonal interactions, unspecified**

d 729   General interpersonal interactions, other specified and unspecified

Particular interpersonal relationships (d730–d779)

d 730   **Relating with strangers**
Engaging in temporary contacts and links with strangers for specific purposes, such as when asking for information, directions or making a purchase.

d 740   **Formal relationships**
Creating and maintaining specific relationships in formal settings, such as with teachers, employers, professionals or service providers.

Inclusions: relating with persons in authority, with subordinates and with equals

> **d 7400   Relating with persons in authority**
> Creating and maintaining formal relations with people in positions of power or of a higher rank or prestige relative to one's own social position, such as an employer.

> **d 7401   Relating with subordinates**
> Creating and maintaining formal relations with people in positions of lower rank or prestige relative to one's own social position, such as an employee or servant.

> **d 7402   Relating with equals**
> Creating and maintaining formal relations with people in the same position of authority, rank or prestige relative to one's own social position.

> **d 7408   Formal relationships, other specified**

d 7409 Formal relationships, unspecified

d 750 Informal social relationships

Entering into relationships with others, such as casual relationships with people living in the same community or residence, or with co-workers, students, playmates or people with similar backgrounds or professions.

Inclusions: informal relationships with friends, neighbours, acquaintances, co-inhabitants and peers

d 7500 Informal relationships with friends

Creating and maintaining friendship relationships that are characterized by mutual esteem and common interests.

d 7501 Informal relationships with neighbours

Creating and maintaining informal relationships with people who live in nearby dwellings or living areas.

d 7502 Informal relationships with acquaintances

Creating and maintaining informal relationships with people whom one knows but who are not close friends.

d 7503 Informal relationships with co-inhabitants

Creating and maintaining informal relationships with people who are co-inhabitants of a house or other dwelling, privately or publicly run, for any purpose.

d 7504 Informal relationships with peers

Creating and maintaining informal relationships with people who share the same age, interest or other common feature.

d 7508 Informal social relationships, other specified

d 7509 Informal social relationships, unspecified

d 760 Family relationships

Creating and maintaining kinship relationships, such as with members of the nuclear family, extended family, foster and adopted family and step-relationships, more distant relationships such as second cousins, or legal guardians.

Inclusions: parent-child and child-parent relationships, sibling and extended family relationships

d 7600   Parent-child relationships
Becoming and being a parent, both natural and adoptive, such as by having a child and relating to it as a parent or creating and maintaining a parental relationship with an adoptive child, and providing physical, intellectual and emotional nurture to one's natural or adoptive child.

d 7601   Child-parent relationships
Creating and maintaining relationships with one's parent, such as a young child obeying his or her parents or an adult child taking care of his or her elderly parents.

d 7602   Sibling relationships
Creating and maintaining a brotherly or sisterly relationship with a person who shares one or both parents by birth, adoption or marriage.

d 7603   Extended family relationships
Creating and maintaining a family relationship with members of one's extended family, such as with cousins, aunts and uncles and grandparents.

d 7608   Family relationships, other specified

d 7609   Family relationships, unspecified

d 770   Intimate relationships
Creating and maintaining close or romantic relationships between individuals, such as husband and wife, lovers or sexual partners.

Inclusions: romantic, spousal and sexual relationships

d 7700   Romantic relationships
Creating and maintaining a relationship based on emotional and physical attraction, potentially leading to long-term intimate relationships.

d 7701   Spousal relationships
Creating and maintaining an intimate relationship of a legal nature with another person, such as in a legal marriage, including becoming and being a legally married wife or husband or an unmarried spouse.

d 7702   Sexual relationships
Creating and maintaining a relationship of a sexual nature, with a spouse or other partner.

d 7708   Intimate relationships, other specified

d 7709   Intimate relationships, unspecified

d 779   Particular interpersonal relationships, other specified and unspecified

d 798   Interpersonal interactions and relationships, other specified

d 799   Interpersonal interactions and relationships, unspecified

Chapter 8

Major life areas

This chapter is about carrying out the tasks and actions required to engage in education, work and employment and to conduct economic transactions.

Education (d810-d839)

d 810   **Informal education**
Learning at home or in some other non-institutional setting, such as acquiring non-academic (e.g. crafts) or academic (e.g. home-schooling) skills from parents or family member in home or community.

d 815   **Preschool education**
Learning at an initial level of organized instruction in the home or in the community designed primarily to introduce a child to a school-type environment and prepare the child for compulsory education, such as by acquiring skills in a day-care or similar setting in preparation for school (e.g. educational services provided in the home or in community settings designed to promote health and cognitive, motor, language and social development and readiness skills for formal education).

> **d 8150**   **Moving into preschool educational programme or across levels**
> Performing activities involved in gaining access to preschool education.
>
> **d 8151**   **Maintaining preschool educational programme**
> Performing activities involved in maintaining participation in preschool education programme activities, such as attending classes, interacting appropriately with peers and teachers, and fulfilling the duties and requirements of being a student.
>
> **d 8152**   **Progressing in preschool educational programme**
> Performing activities involved in completing a programme requirement or another evaluation process relevant to obtaining a preschool education.
>
> **d 8153**   **Terminating preschool educational programme**
> Leaving preschool educational programme in an appropriate manner to enter the next level of school education.
>
> **d 8158**   **Preschool education, other specified**
>
> **d 8159**   **Preschool education, unspecified**

d 816 **Preschool life and related activities**
Engaging in preschool life and related activities, such as excursions and celebrations.

d 820 **School education**
Gaining admission to school, education; engaging in all school-related responsibilities and privileges; learning the course material, subjects and other curriculum requirements in a primary or secondary education programme, including attending school regularly; working cooperatively with other students, taking direction from teachers, organizing, studying and completing assigned tasks and projects, and advancing to other stages of education.

> **d 8200** **Moving into educational programme or across levels**
> Performing activities involved in gaining access to school and transitioning from one stage of school to another.

> **d 8201** **Maintaining educational programme**
> Performing activities involved in maintaining participation in school and school activities, such as attending classes, interacting appropriately with peers and teachers, and fulfilling the duties and requirements of being a student.

> **d 8202** **Progressing in educational programme**
> Performing activities involved in completing a course requirement, exam or another evaluation process relevant to obtaining an education.

> **d 8203** **Terminating educational programme or school levels**
> Leaving school in an appropriate manner to enter the next level of school education, work, employment or other domains of adult life.

> **d 8208** **School education, other specified**

> **d 8209** **School education, unspecified**

d 825 **Vocational training**
Engaging in all activities of a vocational programme and learning the curriculum material in preparation for employment in a trade, job or profession.

> **d 8250** **Moving into vocational training programme or across levels**
> Performing activities involved in gaining access to vocational training and transitioning from one stage of vocational training to another.

> **d 8251** **Maintaining vocational training programme**
> Performing activities involved in maintaining participation in vocational training activities, such as attending classes, interacting appropriately

with peers and teachers, and fulfilling the duties and requirements of being a student.

d 8252 **Progressing in vocational training programme**
Performing activities involved in completing a course requirement, exam or another evaluation process relevant to obtaining vocational training.

d 8253 **Terminating vocational training programme**
Leaving vocational training programme in an appropriate manner to enter the next level of school education, work, employment or other domains of adult life.

d 8258 **Vocational training, other specified**

d 8259 **Vocational training, unspecified**

d 830 **Higher education**
Engaging in the activities of advanced educational programmes in universities, colleges and professional schools and learning all aspects of the curriculum required for degrees, diplomas, certificates and other accreditations, such as completing a university bachelor's or master's course of study, medical school or other professional school.

d 8300 **Moving into higher education or across levels**
Performing activities involved in gaining access to higher education and transitioning from one stage of higher education to another.

d 8301 **Maintaining higher education programme**
Performing activities involved in maintaining participation in higher education activities, such as attending classes, interacting appropriately with peers and teachers, and fulfilling the duties and requirements of being a student.

d 8302 **Progressing in higher education programme**
Performing activities involved in completing a course requirement, exam or another evaluation process relevant to obtaining higher education.

d 8303 **Terminating higher education programme**
Leaving higher education in an appropriate manner to enter the next level of school education, work, employment or other domains of adult life.

d 8308 **Higher education, other specified**

d 8309 **Higher education, unspecified**

d 835 **School life and related activities**
Engaging in aspects of school life and school-related associations, such as student council and student officer.

d 839 **Education, other specified and unspecified**

Work and employment (d840-d859)

d 840 **Apprenticeship (work preparation)**
Engaging in programmes related to preparation for employment, such as performing the tasks required of an apprenticeship, internship, articling and in-service training.

Exclusion: vocational training (d825)

d 845 **Acquiring, keeping and terminating a job**
Seeking, finding and choosing employment, being hired and accepting employment, maintaining and advancing through a job, trade, occupation or profession, and leaving a job in an appropriate manner.

Inclusions: seeking employment; preparing a resume or curriculum vitae; contacting employers and preparing interviews; maintaining a job; monitoring one's own work performance; giving notice; and terminating a job

> **d 8450** **Seeking employment**
> Locating and choosing a job, in a trade, profession or other form of employment, and performing the required tasks to get hired, such as showing up at the place of employment or participating in a job interview.

> **d 8451** **Maintaining a job**
> Performing job-related tasks to keep an occupation, trade, profession or other form of employment, and obtaining promotion and other advancements in employment.

> **d 8452** **Terminating a job**
> Leaving or quitting a job in the appropriate manner.

> **d 8458** **Acquiring, keeping and terminating a job, other specified**

> **d 8459** **Acquiring, keeping and terminating a job, unspecified**

d 850 **Remunerative employment**
Engaging in all aspects of work, as an occupation, trade, profession or other form of employment, for payment, as an employee, full or part time, or self-employed, such as seeking employment and getting a job, doing the required tasks of the job,

attending work on time as required, supervising other workers or being supervised, and performing required tasks alone or in groups.

Inclusions: self-employment, part-time and full-time employment

d 8500   Self-employment
Engaging in remunerative work sought or generated by the individual, or contracted from others without a formal employment relationship, such as migratory agricultural work, working as a free-lance writer or consultant, short-term contract work, working as an artist or crafts person, owning and running a shop or other business.

Exclusions: part-time and full-time employment (d8501, d8502)

d 8501   Part-time employment
Engaging in all aspects of work for payment on a part-time basis, as an employee, such as seeking employment and getting a job, doing the tasks required of the job, attending work on time as required, supervising other workers or being supervised, and performing required tasks alone or in groups.

d 8502   Full-time employment
Engaging in all aspects of work for payment on a full-time basis, as an employee, such as seeking employment and getting a job, doing the required tasks of the job, attending work on time as required, supervising other workers or being supervised, and performing required tasks alone or in groups.

d 8508   Remunerative employment, other specified

d 8509   Remunerative employment, unspecified

d 855   Non-remunerative employment
Engaging in all aspects of work in which pay is not provided, full-time or part-time, including organized work activities, doing the required tasks of the job, attending work on time as required, supervising other workers or being supervised, and performing required tasks alone or in groups, such as volunteer work, charity work, working for a community or religious group without remuneration, working around the home without remuneration.

Exclusion: Chapter 6 Domestic Life

d 859   Work and employment, other specified and unspecified

Economic life (d860-d879)

d 860 **Basic economic transactions**
Engaging in any form of simple economic transaction, such as using money to purchase food or bartering, exchanging goods or services; or saving money.

d 865 **Complex economic transactions**
Engaging in any form of complex economic transaction that involves the exchange of capital or property, and the creation of profit or economic value, such as buying a business, factory, or equipment, maintaining a bank account, or trading in commodities.

d 870 **Economic self-sufficiency**
Having command over economic resources, from private or public sources, in order to ensure economic security for present and future needs.

Inclusions: personal economic resources and public economic entitlements

d 8700 **Personal economic resources**
Having command over personal or private economic resources, in order to ensure economic security for present and future needs.

d 8701 **Public economic entitlements**
Having command over public economic resources, in order to ensure economic security for present and future needs.

d 8708 **Economic self-sufficiency, other specified**

d 8709 **Economic self-sufficiency, unspecified**

d 879 **Economic life, other specified and unspecified**

d 880 **Engagement in play**
Purposeful, sustained engagement in activities with objects, toys, materials or games, occupying oneself or with others.

d 8800 **Solitary play**
Occupying oneself in purposeful, sustained engagement in activities with objects, toys, materials or games.

d 8801 **Onlooker play**
Occupying oneself by purposeful observation of the activities of others with objects, toys, materials or games, but not joining in their activities.

d 8802   Parallel play
Engaging in purposeful, sustained activities with objects, toys, materials or games in the presence of other persons also engaged in play, but not joining in their activities.

d 8803   Shared cooperative play
Joining others in sustained engagement in activities with objects, toys, materials or games with a shared goal or purpose.

d 8808   Engagement in play, other specified

d 8809   Engagement in play, unspecified

d 898   **Major life areas, other specified**

d 899   **Major life areas, unspecified**

Chapter 9

Community, social and civic life

This chapter is about the actions and tasks required to engage in organized social life outside the family, in community, social and civic areas of life.

d 910 **Community life**
Engaging in aspects of community social life, such as engaging in charitable organizations, service clubs or professional social organizations.

Inclusions: informal and formal associations; ceremonies

Exclusions: non-remunerative employment (d855); recreation and leisure (d920); religion and spirituality (d930); political life and citizenship (d950)

> **d 9100** **Informal associations**
> Engaging in social or community associations organized by people with common interests, such as local social clubs or ethnic groups.

> **d 9101** **Formal associations**
> Engaging in professional or other exclusive social groups, such as associations of lawyers, physicians or academics.

> **d 9102** **Ceremonies**
> Engaging in non-religious rites or social ceremonies, such as marriages, funerals or initiation ceremonies.

> **d 9103** **Informal community life**
> Engaging in communal gatherings with others at playgrounds, parks, street cafes, town squares and other common public spaces.

> **d 9108** **Community life, other specified**

> **d 9109** **Community life, unspecified**

d 920 **Recreation and leisure**
Engaging in any form of play, recreational or leisure activity, such as informal or organized play and sports, programmes of physical fitness, relaxation, amusement or diversion, going to art galleries, museums, cinemas or theatres; engaging in crafts or hobbies, reading for enjoyment, playing musical instruments; sightseeing, tourism and travelling for pleasure.

Inclusions: games, sports, arts and culture, crafts, hobbies and socializing

Exclusions: riding animals for transportation (d480); remunerative and non-remunerative work (d850 and d855); engagement in play (d880); religion and spirituality (d930); political life and citizenship (d950)

d 9200   Play
Engaging in games with rules or unstructured or unorganized games and spontaneous recreation, such as playing chess or cards, board games or activities with a set of rules (e.g. hide-and-seek).

Exclusion: engagement in play (d880)

d 9201   Sports
Engaging in competitive and informal or formally organized games or athletic events, performed alone or in a group, such as bowling, gymnastics or soccer.

d 9202   Arts and culture
Engaging in, or appreciating, fine arts or cultural events, such as going to the theatre, cinema, museum or art gallery, or acting in a play, dancing, being read to or reading for enjoyment, singing in a group or playing a musical instrument.

d 9203   Crafts
Engaging in handicrafts, such as pottery, knitting or working with wood to make toys or other objects.

d 9204   Hobbies
Engaging in pastimes, such as collecting stamps, coins, antiques, stones, shells or pictures.

d 9205   Socializing
Engaging in informal or casual gatherings with others, such as visiting friends or relatives or meeting informally in public places.

d 9208   Recreation and leisure, other specified

d 9209   Recreation and leisure, unspecified

d 930   Religion and spirituality
Engaging in religious or spiritual activities, organizations and practices for self-fulfilment, finding meaning, religious or spiritual value and establishing connection with a divine power, such as is involved in attending a church, temple, mosque or synagogue, praying or chanting for a religious purpose, and spiritual contemplation.

Inclusions: organized religion and spirituality

d 9300   Organized religion
Engaging in organized religious ceremonies, activities and events.

d 9301   Spirituality
Engaging in spiritual activities or events, outside an organized religion.

d 9308   Religion and spirituality, other specified

d 9309   Religion and spirituality, unspecified

d 940   Human rights
Enjoying all nationally and internationally recognized rights that are accorded to people by virtue of their humanity alone, such as human rights as recognized by the United Nations Universal Declaration of Human Rights (1948) and the United Nations Standard Rules for the Equalization of Opportunities for Persons with Disabilities (1993); the United Nations Convention on the Rights of the Child (1989); the right to self-determination or autonomy; and the right to control over one's destiny.

Exclusion: political life and citizenship (d950)

d 950   Political life and citizenship
Engaging in the social, political and governmental life of a citizen, having legal status as a citizen and enjoying the rights, protections, privileges and duties associated with that role, such as the right to vote and run for political office, to form political associations; enjoying the rights and freedoms associated with citizenship (e.g. the rights of freedom of speech, association, religion, protection against unreasonable search and seizure, the right to counsel, to a trial and other legal rights and protection against discrimination); having legal standing as a citizen.

Exclusion: human rights (d940)

d 998   Community, social and civic life, other specified

d 999   Community, social and civic life, unspecified

ENVIRONMENTAL FACTORS

Definition: *Environmental factors make up the physical, social and attitudinal environment in which people live and conduct their lives.*

Coding environmental factors

Environmental Factors is a component of Part 2 (Contextual factors) of the classification. These factors must be considered for each component of functioning and coded accordingly (see Annex 2).

Environmental factors are to be coded from the perspective of the person whose situation is being described. For example, kerb cuts without textured paving may be coded as a facilitator for a wheelchair user but as a barrier for a blind person.

The first qualifier indicates the extent to which a factor is a facilitator or a barrier. There are several reasons why an environmental factor may be a facilitator or a barrier, and to what extent. For facilitators, the coder should keep in mind issues such as the accessibility of a resource, and whether access is dependable or variable, of good or poor quality, and so on. In the case of barriers, it might be relevant how often a factor hinders the person, whether the hindrance is great or small, or avoidable or not. It should also be kept in mind that an environmental factor can be a barrier either because of its presence (for example, negative attitudes towards people with disabilities) or its absence (for example, the unavailability of a needed service). The effects that environmental factors have on the lives of people with health conditions are varied and complex, and it is hoped that future research will lead to better understanding of this interaction and, possibly, show the usefulness of a second qualifier for these factors.

In some instances, a diverse collection of environmental factors is summarized with a single term, such as poverty, development, rural or urban setting or social capital. These summary terms are not themselves found in the classification. Rather, the coder should separate the constituent factors and code these. Once again, further research is required to determine whether there are clear and consistent sets of environmental factors that make up each of these summary terms.

First qualifier

The following is the negative and positive scale for the extent to which an environmental factor acts as a barrier or a facilitator. A point or separator alone denotes a barrier, and the + sign denotes a facilitator, as indicated below:

xxx.0 NO barrier	(none, absent, negligible,...)	0-4%
xxx.1 MILD barrier	(slight, low,...)	5-24%
xxx.2 MODERATE barrier	(medium, fair,...)	25-49%
xxx.3 SEVERE barrier	(high, extreme, ...)	50-95%
xxx.4 COMPLETE barrier	(total,...)	96-100%
xxx+0 NO facilitator	(none, absent, negligible,...)	0-4%
xxx+1 MILD facilitator	(slight, low,...)	5-24%

xxx+2	MODERATE facilitator	(medium, fair,...)	25-49%
xxx+3	SUBSTANTIAL facilitator	(high, extreme, …)	50-95%
xxx+4	COMPLETE facilitator	(total,…)	96-100%
xxx.8	barrier, not specified		
xxx+8	facilitator, not specified		
xxx.9	not applicable		

Broad ranges of percentages are provided for those cases in which calibrated assessment instruments or other standards are available to quantify the extent of the barrier or facilitator in the environment. For example, when "no barrier" or a "complete barrier" is coded, this scaling has a margin of error of up to 5%. A "moderate barrier" is defined as up to half of the scale of a total barrier. The percentages are to be calibrated in different domains with reference to population standards as percentiles. For this quantification to be used in a uniform manner, assessment procedures have to be developed through research.

Second qualifier: To be developed.

Chapter 1

Products and technology

This chapter is about the natural or human-made products or systems of products, equipment and technology in an individual's immediate environment that are gathered, created, produced or manufactured. The ISO 9999 classification of technical aids defines these as "any product, instrument, equipment or technical system used by a disabled person, especially produced or generally available, preventing, compensating, monitoring, relieving or neutralizing" disability. It is recognized that any product or technology can be assistive. (See ISO 9999: Technical aids for disabled persons - Classification (second version); ISO/TC 173/SC 2; ISO/DIS 9999 (rev.).) For the purposes of this classification of environmental factors, however, assistive products and technology are defined more narrowly as any product, instrument, equipment or technology adapted or specially designed for improving the functioning of a disabled person.

e110 **Products or substances for personal consumption**
Any natural or human-made object or substance gathered, processed or manufactured for ingestion.

Inclusions: food (including breast milk), drink and drugs

> **e1100** **Food**
> Any natural or human-made object or substance gathered, processed or manufactured for consumption, such as raw, processed and prepared food and liquids of different consistencies, herbs and minerals (vitamin and other supplements).

> **e1101** **Drugs**
> Any natural or human-made object or substance gathered, processed or manufactured for medicinal purposes, such as allopathic and naturopathic medication.

> **e1108** **Products or substances for personal consumption, other specified**

> **e1109** **Products or substances for personal consumption, unspecified**

e115 **Products and technology for personal use in daily living**
Equipment, products and technologies used by people in daily activities, including those adapted or specially designed, located in, on or near the person using them.

Inclusions: general and assistive products and technology for personal use

Exclusions: products and technology for personal indoor and outdoor mobility and transportation (e120); products and technology for communication (e125)

e 1150 **General products and technology for personal use in daily living**
Equipment, products and technologies used by people in their daily activities, such as clothes, textiles, furniture, appliances, cleaning products and tools, not adapted or specially designed, except as appropriate for age, such as utensils for children.

e 1151 **Assistive products and technology for personal use in daily living**
Adapted or specially designed equipment, products and technologies that assist people in daily living, such as prosthetic and orthotic devices, neural prostheses (e.g. functional stimulation devices that control bowels, bladder, breathing and heart rate), and environmental control units aimed at facilitating individuals' control over their indoor setting (scanners, remote control systems, voice-controlled systems, timer switches).

e 1152 **Products and technology used for play**
Equipment, products and technologies used in structured or unstructured play by an individual or group, not adapted or specially designed, except as appropriate for age.

Exclusions: general products and technology for personal use in daily living (e1150); assistive products and technology for personal use in daily living (e1151); products and technology for education (e130); products and technology for culture, recreation and sport (e140)

　　e 11520 **General products and technology for play**
Objects, material, toys and other products used in play such as blocks, balls, miniature objects, games, puzzles, swings and slides.

　　e 11521 **Adapted products and technology for play**
Objects, material, toys and other products adapted or specially designed to assist play, such as remote control cars and modified playground equipment.

　　e 11528 **Products and technology used for play, other specified**

　　e 11529 **Products and technology used for play, unspecified**

e 1158 **Products and technology for personal use in daily living, other specified**

e 1159 **Products and technology for personal use in daily living, unspecified**

e 120 **Products and technology for personal indoor and outdoor mobility and transportation**
Equipment, products and technologies used by people in activities of moving inside and outside buildings, including those adapted or specially designed, located in, on or near the person using them.

Inclusions: general and assistive products and technology for personal indoor and outdoor mobility and transportation

    e 1200 **General products and technology for personal indoor and outdoor mobility and transportation**
Equipment, products and technologies used by people in activities of moving inside and outside buildings, such as motorized and non-motorized vehicles used for the transportation of people over ground, water and air (e.g. buses, cars, vans, other motor-powered vehicles and animal-powered transporters), not adapted or specially designed, except as appropriate for age, such as tricycles and prams.

    e 1201 **Assistive products and technology for personal indoor and outdoor mobility and transportation**
Adapted or specially designed equipment, products and technologies that assist people to move inside and outside buildings, such as walking devices, special cars and vans, adaptations to vehicles, wheelchairs, scooters and transfer devices.

    e 1208 **Products and technology for personal indoor and outdoor mobility and transportation, other specified**

    e 1209 **Products and technology for personal indoor and outdoor mobility and transportation, unspecified**

e 125 **Products and technology for communication**
Equipment, products and technologies used by people in activities of sending and receiving information, including those adapted or specially designed, located in, on or near the person using them.

Inclusions: general and assistive products and technology for communication

    e 1250 **General products and technology for communication**
Equipment, products and technologies used by people in activities of sending and receiving information, such as optical and auditory devices, audio recorders and receivers, television and video equipment, telephone devices, sound transmission systems and face-to-face communication devices, not adapted or specially designed.

e 1251   Assistive products and technology for communication
Adapted or specially designed equipment, products and technologies that assist people to send and receive information, such as specialized vision devices, electro-optical devices, specialized writing devices, drawing or handwriting devices, signalling systems and special computer software and hardware, cochlear implants, hearing aids, FM auditory trainers, voice prostheses, communication boards, glasses and contact lenses.

e 1258   Products and technology for communication, other specified

e 1259   Products and technology for communication, unspecified

e 130   **Products and technology for education**
Equipment, products, processes, methods and technology used for acquisition of knowledge, expertise or skill, including those adapted or specially designed.

Inclusions: general and assistive products and technology for education

e 1300   General products and technology for education
Equipment, products, processes, methods and technology used for acquisition of knowledge, expertise or skill at any level, such as books, manuals, educational toys, computer hardware or software, not adapted or specially designed.

e 1301   Assistive products and technology for education
Adapted and specially designed equipment, products, processes, methods and technology used for acquisition of knowledge, expertise or skill, such as specialized computer technology.

e 1308   Products and technology for education, other specified

e 1309   Products and technology for education, unspecified

e 135   **Products and technology for employment**
Equipment, products and technology used for employment to facilitate work activities.

Inclusions: general and assistive products and technology for employment

e 1350   General products and technology for employment
Equipment, products and technology used for employment to facilitate work activities, such as tools, machines and office equipment, not adapted or specially designed.

e 1351   Assistive products and technology for employment
Adapted or specially designed equipment, products and technology used for employment to facilitate work activities, such as adjustable tables, desks and filing cabinets; remote control entry and exit of office doors; computer hardware, software, accessories and environmental control units aimed at facilitating an individual's conduct of work-related tasks and aimed at control of the work environment (e.g. scanners, remote control systems, voice-controlled systems and timer switches).

e 1358   Products and technology for employment, other specified

e 1359   Products and technology for employment, unspecified

e 140   Products and technology for culture, recreation and sport
Equipment, products and technology used for the conduct and enhancement of cultural, recreational and sporting activities, including those adapted or specially designed.

Inclusions: general and assistive products and technology for culture, recreation and sport

Exclusion: products and technology for play (e1152)

e 1400   General products and technology for culture, recreation and sport
Equipment, products and technology used for the conduct and enhancement of cultural, recreational and sporting activities, such as toys, skis, tennis balls and musical instruments, not adapted or specially designed.

e 1401   Assistive products and technology for culture, recreation and sport
Adapted or specially designed equipment, products and technology used for the conduct and enhancement of cultural, recreational and sporting activities, such as modified mobility devices for sports, adaptations for musical and other artistic performance.

e 1408   Products and technology for culture, recreation and sport, other specified

e 1409   Products and technology for culture, recreation and sport, unspecified

e 145   Products and technology for the practice of religion and spirituality
Products and technology, unique or mass-produced, that are given or take on a symbolic meaning in the context of the practice of religion or spirituality, including those adapted or specially designed.

Inclusions: general and assistive products and technology for the practice of religion and spirituality

e 1450 **General products and technology for the practice of religion or spirituality**
Products and technology, unique or mass-produced, that are given or take on a symbolic meaning in the context of the practice of religion or spirituality, such as spirit houses, maypoles, headdresses, masks, crucifixes, menorahs and prayer mats, not adapted or specially designed, except as appropriate for age.

e 1451 **Assistive products and technology for the practice of religion or spirituality**
Adapted or specially designed products and technology that are given, or take on a symbolic meaning in the context of the practice of religion or spirituality, such as Braille religious books, Braille tarot cards, and special protection for wheelchair wheels when entering temples.

e 1458 **Products and technology for the practice of religion or spirituality, other specified**

e 1459 **Products and technology for the practice of religion or spirituality, unspecified**

e 150 **Design, construction and building products and technology of buildings for public use**
Products and technology that constitute an individual's indoor and outdoor human-made environment that is planned, designed and constructed for public use, including those adapted or specially designed.

Inclusions: design, construction and building products and technology of entrances and exits, facilities and routing

e 1500 **Design, construction and building products and technology for entering and exiting buildings for public use**
Products and technology of entry and exit from the human-made environment that is planned, designed and constructed for public use, such as design, building and construction of entries and exits to buildings for public use (e.g. workplaces, shops and theatres), public buildings, portable and stationary ramps, power-assisted doors, lever door handles and level door thresholds.

e 1501 **Design, construction and building products and technology for gaining access to facilities inside buildings for public use**
Products and technology of indoor facilities in design, building and construction for public use, such as washroom facilities, telephones,

audio loops, lifts or elevators, escalators, thermostats (for temperature regulation) and dispersed accessible seating in auditoriums or stadiums.

e 1502   Design, construction and building products and technology for way finding, path routing and designation of locations in buildings for public use
Indoor and outdoor products and technology in design, building and construction for public use to assist people to find their way inside and immediately outside buildings and locate the places they want to go to, such as signage, in Braille or writing, size of corridors, floor surfaces, accessible kiosks and other forms of directories.

e 1503   Design, construction and building products and technology for physical safety of persons in buildings for public use
Indoor and outdoor products and technology for public use to assure safety, such as guardrails for beds and emergency signals.

e 1508   Design, construction and building products and technology of buildings for public use, other specified

e 1509   Design, construction and building products and technology of buildings for public use, unspecified

e 155   Design, construction and building products and technology of buildings for private use
Products and technology that constitute an individual's indoor and outdoor human-made environment that is planned, designed and constructed for private use (e.g. home, dwelling), including those adapted or specially designed.

Inclusions: design, construction and building products and technology of entrances and exits, facilities and routing

e 1550   Design, construction and building products and technology for entering and exiting of buildings for private use
Products and technology of entry and exit from the human-made environment that is planned, designed and constructed for private use, such as entries and exits to private homes, portable and stationary ramps, power-assisted doors, lever door handles and level door thresholds.

e 1551   Design, construction and building products and technology for gaining access to facilities in buildings for private use
Products and technology related to design, building and construction inside buildings for private use, such as washroom facilities, telephones, audio loops, kitchen cabinets, appliances and electronic controls in private homes.

e 1552 **Design, construction and building products and technology for way finding, path routing and designation of locations in buildings for private use**
Indoor and outdoor products and technology in the design, building and construction of path routing, for private use, to assist people to find their way inside and immediately outside buildings and locate the places they want to go to, such as signage, in Braille or writing, size of corridors and floor surfaces.

e 1553 **Design, construction and building products and technology for physical safety of persons in buildings for private use**
Indoor and outdoor products and technology for private use to assure safety, such as guardrails, emergency signals and secure storage of hazardous objects (e.g. weapons) or materials (e.g. solvents, insecticides).

e 1558 **Design, construction and building products and technology of buildings for private use, other specified**

e 1559 **Design, construction and building products and technology of buildings for private use, unspecified**

e 160 **Products and technology of land development**
Products and technology of land areas, as they affect an individual's outdoor environment through the implementation of land use policies, design, planning and development of space, including those adapted or specially designed.

Inclusions: products and technology of land areas that have been organized by the implementation of land use policies, such as rural areas, suburban areas, urban areas, parks, conservation areas and wildlife reserves

e 1600 **Products and technology of rural land development**
Products and technology in rural land areas, as they affect an individual's outdoor environment through the implementation of rural land use policies, design, planning and development of space, such as farm lands, pathways and signposting.

e 1601 **Products and technology of suburban land development**
Products and technology in suburban land areas, as they affect an individual's outdoor environment through the implementation of suburban land use policies, design, planning and development of space, such as kerb cuts, pathways, signposting and street lighting.

e 1602 **Products and technology of urban land development**
Products and technology in urban land areas as they affect an individual's outdoor environment through the implementation of urban land use policies, design, planning and development of space, such as kerb cuts,

ramps, signposting and street lighting.

e 1603   Products and technology of parks, conservation and wildlife areas
Products and technology in land areas making up parks, conservation and wildlife areas, as they affect an individual's outdoor environment through the implementation of land use policies and design, planning and development of space, such as park signage and wildlife trails.

e 1608   Products and technology of land development, other specified

e 1609   Products and technology of land development, unspecified

e 165   Assets
Products or objects of economic exchange such as money, goods, property and other valuables that an individual owns or of which he or she has rights of use or rights of benefit, such as child support payment or wills for children or dependent persons.

Inclusions: tangible and intangible products and goods, financial assets

e 1650   Financial assets
Products, such as money and other financial instruments, which serve as a medium of exchange for labour, capital goods and services.

e 1651   Tangible assets
Products or objects, such as houses and land, clothing, food and technical goods, which serve as a medium of exchange for labour, capital goods and services.

e 1652   Intangible assets
Products, such as intellectual property, knowledge and skills, which serve as a medium of exchange for labour, capital goods and services.

e 1658   Assets, other specified

e 1659   Assets, unspecified

e 198   Products and technology, other specified

e 199   Products and technology, unspecified

Chapter 2

Natural environment and human-made changes to environment

This chapter is about animate and inanimate elements of the natural or physical environment, and components of that environment that have been modified by people, as well as characteristics of human populations within that environment.

e 210   **Physical geography**
Features of land forms and bodies of water.

Inclusions: features of geography included within orography (relief, quality and expanse of land and land forms, including altitude) and hydrography (bodies of water such as lakes, rivers, sea)

e 2100   **Land forms**
Features of land forms, such as mountains, hills, valleys and plains.

e 2101   **Bodies of water**
Features of bodies of water, such as lakes, dams, rivers and streams.

e 2108   **Physical geography, other specified**

e 2109   **Physical geography, unspecified**

e 215   **Population**
Groups of people living in a given environment who share the same pattern of environmental adaptation.

Inclusions: demographic change; population density

e 2150   **Demographic change**
Changes occurring within groups of people, such as the composition and variation in the total number of individuals in an area caused by birth, death, ageing of a population and migration.

e 2151   **Population density**
Number of people per unit of land area, including features such as high and low density.

e 2158   **Population, other specified**

e 2159   **Population, unspecified**

e 220   **Flora and fauna**
Plants and animals.

Exclusions: domesticated animals (e350); population (e215)

e 2200   Plants

Any of various photosynthetic, eukaryotic, multicellular organisms of the kingdom Plantae characteristically producing embryos, containing chloroplasts, having cellulose cell walls, and lacking the power of locomotion, such as trees, flowers, shrubs and vines.

e 2201   Animals

Multicellular organisms of the kingdom Animalia, differing from plants in certain typical characteristics such as capacity for locomotion, non-photosynthetic metabolism, pronounced response to stimuli, restricted growth, and fixed bodily structure, such as wild or farm animals, reptiles, birds, fish and mammals.

Exclusions: assets (e165); domesticated animals (e350)

e 2208   Fauna and flora, other specified

e 2209   Fauna and flora, unspecified

e 225   **Climate**
Meteorological features and events, such as the weather.

Inclusions: temperature, humidity, atmospheric pressure, precipitation, wind and seasonal variations

e 2250   Temperature

Degree of heat or cold, such as high and low temperature, normal or extreme temperature.

e 2251   Humidity

Level of moisture in the air, such as high or low humidity.

e 2252   Atmospheric pressure

Pressure of the surrounding air, such as pressure related to height above sea level or meteorological conditions.

e 2253   Precipitation

Falling of moisture, such as rain, dew, snow, sleet and hail.

e 2254   **Wind**
Air in more or less rapid natural motion, such as a breeze, gale or gust.

e 2255   **Seasonal variation**
Natural, regular and predictable changes from one season to the next, such as summer, autumn, winter and spring.

e 2258   **Climate, other specified**

e 2259   **Climate, unspecified**

e 230   Natural events
Geographic and atmospheric changes that cause disruption in an individual's physical environment, occurring regularly or irregularly, such as earthquakes and severe or violent weather conditions, e.g. tornadoes, hurricanes, typhoons, floods, forest fires and ice-storms.

e 235   Human-caused events
Alterations or disturbances in the natural environment, caused by humans, that may result in the disruption of people's day-to-day lives, including events or conditions linked to conflict and wars, such as the displacement of people, destruction of social infrastructure, homes and lands, environmental disasters and land, water or air pollution (e.g. toxic spills).

e 240   Light
Electromagnetic radiation by which things are made visible by either sunlight or artificial lighting (e.g. candles, oil or paraffin lamps, fires and electricity), and which may provide useful or distracting information about the world.

Inclusions: light intensity; light quality; colour contrasts

e 2400   **Light intensity**
Level or amount of energy being emitted by either a natural (e.g. sun) or an artificial source of light.

e 2401   **Light quality**
The nature of the light being provided and related colour contrasts created in the visual surroundings, and which may provide useful information about the world (e.g. visual information on the presence of stairs or a door) or distractions (e.g. too many visual images).

e 2408   **Light, other specified**

e 2409   **Light, unspecified**

e 245 **Time-related changes**
Natural, regular or predictable temporal change.

Inclusions: day/night and lunar cycles

e 2450 **Day/night cycles**
Natural, regular and predictable changes from day through to night and back to day, such as day, night, dawn and dusk.

e 2451 **Lunar cycles**
Natural, regular and predictable changes of the moon's position in relation to the earth.

e 2458 **Time-related changes, other specified**

e 2459 **Time-related changes, unspecified**

e 250 **Sound**
A phenomenon that is or may be heard, such as banging, ringing, thumping, singing, whistling, yelling or buzzing, in any volume, timbre or tone, and that may provide useful or distracting information about the world.

Inclusions: sound intensity; sound quality

e 2500 **Sound intensity**
Level or volume of auditory phenomenon determined by the amount of energy being generated, where high energy levels are perceived as loud sounds and low energy levels as soft sounds.

e 2501 **Sound quality**
Nature of a sound as determined by the wavelength and wave pattern of the sound and perceived as the timbre and tone, such as harshness or melodiousness, and which may provide useful information about the world (e.g. sound of dog barking versus a cat miaowing) or distractions (e.g. background noise).

e 2508 **Sound, other specified**

e 2509 **Sound, unspecified**

e 255 **Vibration**
Regular or irregular to and fro motion of an object or an individual caused by a physical disturbance, such as shaking, quivering, quick jerky movements of things, buildings or people caused by small or large equipment, aircraft and explosions.

Exclusion: natural events (e230), such as vibration or shaking of the earth caused by earthquakes

e 260   **Air quality**
Characteristics of the atmosphere (outside buildings) or enclosed areas of air (inside buildings), and which may provide useful or distracting information about the world.

Inclusions: indoor and outdoor air quality

e 2600   **Indoor air quality**
Nature of the air inside buildings or enclosed areas, as determined by odour, smoke, humidity, air conditioning (controlled air quality) or uncontrolled air quality, and which may provide useful information about the world (e.g. smell of leaking gas) or distractions (e.g. overpowering smell of perfume).

e 2601   **Outdoor air quality**
Nature of the air outside buildings or enclosed areas, as determined by odour, smoke, humidity, ozone levels, and other features of the atmosphere, and which may provide useful information about the world (e.g. smell of rain) or distractions (e.g. toxic smells).

e 2608   **Air quality, other specified**

e 2609   **Air quality, unspecified**

e 298   Natural environment and human-made changes to environment, other specified

e 299   Natural environment and human-made changes to environment, unspecified

Chapter 3

Support and relationships

This chapter is about people or animals that provide practical physical or emotional support, nurturing, protection, assistance and relationships to other persons, in their home, place of work, school or at play or in other aspects of their daily activities. The chapter does not encompass the attitudes of the person or people that are providing the support. The environmental factor being described is not the person or animal, but the amount of physical and emotional support the person or animal provides.

e 310   **Immediate family**
Individuals related by birth, marriage or other relationship recognized by the culture as immediate family, such as spouses, partners, parents, siblings, children, foster parents, adoptive parents and grandparents.

Exclusions: extended family (e315); personal care providers and personal assistants (e340)

e 315   **Extended family**
Individuals related through family or marriage or other relationships recognized by the culture as extended family, such as aunts, uncles, nephews and nieces.

Exclusion: immediate family (e310)

e 320   **Friends**
Individuals who are close and ongoing participants in relationships characterized by trust and mutual support.

e 325   **Acquaintances, peers, colleagues, neighbours and community members**
Individuals who are familiar to each other as acquaintances, peers, colleagues, neighbours, and community members, in situations of work, school, recreation, or other aspects of life, and who share demographic features such as age, gender, religious creed or ethnicity or pursue common interests.

Exclusions: associations and organizational services (e5550)

e 330   **People in positions of authority**
Individuals who have decision-making responsibilities for others and who have socially defined influence or power based on their social, economic, cultural or religious roles in society, such as teachers, employers, supervisors, religious leaders, substitute decision-makers, guardians or trustees.

e 335   **People in subordinate positions**
Individuals whose day-to-day life is influenced by people in positions of authority

in work, school or other settings, such as students, workers and members of a religious group.

Exclusion: immediate family (e310)

e 340   **Personal care providers and personal assistants**
Individuals who provide services as required to support individuals in their daily activities and maintenance of performance at work, education or other life situation, provided either through public or private funds, or else on a voluntary basis, such as providers of support for home-making and maintenance, personal assistants, transport assistants, paid help, nannies and others who function as primary caregivers.

Exclusions: immediate family (e310); extended family (e315); friends (e320); general social support services (e5750); health professionals (e355)

e 345   **Strangers**
Individuals who are unfamiliar and unrelated, or those who have not yet established a relationship or association, including persons unknown to the individual but who are sharing a life situation with them, such as substitute teachers co-workers or care providers.

e 350   **Domesticated animals**
Animals that provide physical, emotional, or psychological support, such as pets (dogs, cats, birds, fish, etc.) and animals for personal mobility and transportation.

Exclusions: animals (e2201); assets (e165)

e 355   **Health professionals**
All service providers working within the context of the health system, such as doctors, nurses, physiotherapists, occupational therapists, speech therapists, audiologists, orthotist-prosthetists, medical social workers.

Exclusion: other professionals (e360)

e 360   **Other professionals**
All service providers working outside the health system, including social workers, lawyers, teachers, architects, and designers.

Exclusion: health professionals (e355)

e 398   **Support and relationships, other specified**

e 399   **Support and relationships, unspecified**

Chapter 4

Attitudes

This chapter is about the attitudes that are the observable consequences of customs, practices, ideologies, values, norms, factual beliefs and religious beliefs. These attitudes influence individual behaviour and social life at all levels, from interpersonal relationships and community associations to political, economic and legal structures; for example, individual or societal attitudes about a person's trustworthiness and value as a human being may motivate positive, honorific practices or negative and discriminatory practices (e.g. stigmatizing, stereotyping and marginalizing or neglect of the person). The attitudes classified are those of people external to the person whose situation is being described. They are not those of the person themselves. The individual attitudes are categorized according to the kinds of relationships listed in Environmental Factors Chapter 3. Values and beliefs are not coded separately from attitudes as they are assumed to be the driving forces behind the attitudes.

e 410   **Individual attitudes of immediate family members**
General or specific opinions and beliefs of immediate family members about the person or about other matters (e.g. social, political and economic issues), that influence individual behaviour and actions.

e 415   **Individual attitudes of extended family members**
General or specific opinions and beliefs of extended family members about the person or about other matters (e.g. social, political and economic issues), that influence individual behaviour and actions.

e 420   **Individual attitudes of friends**
General or specific opinions and beliefs of friends about the person or about other matters (e.g. social, political and economic issues), that influence individual behaviour and actions.

e 425   **Individual attitudes of acquaintances, peers, colleagues, neighbours and community members**
General or specific opinions and beliefs of acquaintances, peers, colleagues, neighbours and community members about the person or about other matters (e.g. social, political and economic issues), that influence individual behaviour and actions.

e 430   **Individual attitudes of people in positions of authority**
General or specific opinions and beliefs of people in positions of authority about the person or about other matters (e.g. social, political and economic issues), that influence individual behaviour and actions.

e 435   **Individual attitudes of people in subordinate positions**
General or specific opinions and beliefs of people in subordinate positions about the person or about other matters (e.g. social, political and economic issues), that influence individual behaviour and actions.

e 440   **Individual attitudes of personal care providers and personal assistants**
General or specific opinions and beliefs of personal care providers and personal assistants about the person or about other matters (e.g. social, political and economic issues), that influence individual behaviour and actions.

e 445   **Individual attitudes of strangers**
General or specific opinions and beliefs of strangers about the person or about other matters (e.g. social, political and economic issues), that influence individual behaviour and actions.

e 450   **Individual attitudes of health professionals**
General or specific opinions and beliefs of health professionals about the person or about other matters (e.g. social, political and economic issues), that influence individual behaviour and actions.

e 455   **Individual attitudes of other professionals**
General or specific opinions and beliefs of health-related and other professionals about the person or about other matters (e.g. social, political and economic issues), that influence individual behaviour and actions.

e 460   **Societal attitudes**
General or specific opinions and beliefs generally held by people of a culture, society, subcultural or other social group about other individuals or about other social, political and economic issues, that influence group or individual behaviour and actions.

e 465   **Social norms, practices and ideologies**
Customs, practices, rules and abstract systems of values and normative beliefs (e.g. ideologies, normative world views and moral philosophies) that arise within social contexts and that affect or create societal and individual practices and behaviours, such as social norms of moral and religious behaviour or etiquette; religious doctrine and resulting norms and practices; norms governing rituals or social gatherings.

e 498   **Attitudes, other specified**

e 499   **Attitudes, unspecified**

Chapter 5

Services, systems and policies

This chapter is about:

1. *Services* that provide benefits, structured programmes and operations, in various sectors of society, designed to meet the needs of individuals. (Included in services are the people who provide them.) Services may be public, private or voluntary, and may be established at a local, community, regional, state, provincial, national or international level by individuals, associations, organizations, agencies or governments. The goods provided by these services may be general or adapted and specially designed.

2. *Systems* that are administrative control and organizational mechanisms, and are established by governments at the local, regional, national, and international levels, or by other recognized authorities. These systems are designed to organize, control and monitor services that provide benefits, structured programmes and operations in various sectors of society.

3. *Policies* constituted by rules, regulations, conventions and standards established by governments at the local, regional, national, and international levels, or by other recognized authorities. Policies govern and regulate the systems that organize, control and monitor services, structured programmes and operations in various sectors of society.

e 510 **Services, systems and policies for the production of consumer goods**
Services, systems and policies that govern and provide for the production of objects and products consumed or used by people.

> **e 5100** **Services for the production of consumer goods**
> Services and programmes for the collection, creation, production and manufacturing of consumer goods and products, such as for products and technology used for mobility, communication, education, transportation, employment and housework, including those who provide these services.
>
> *Exclusions: education and training services (e5850); communication services (e5350); Chapter 1*

> **e 5101** **Systems for the production of consumer goods**
> Administrative control and monitoring mechanisms, such as regional, national or international organizations that set standards (e.g. International Organization for Standardization) and consumer bodies, that govern the collection, creation, production and manufacturing of consumer goods and products.

e 5102 **Policies for the production of consumer goods**
Legislation, regulations and standards for the collection, creation, production and manufacturing of consumer goods and products, such as which standards to adopt.

e 5108 **Services, systems and policies for the production of consumer goods, other specified**

e 5109 **Services, systems and policies for the production of consumer goods, unspecified**

e 515 **Architecture and construction services, systems and policies**
Services, systems and policies for the design and construction of buildings, public and private.

Exclusion: open space planning services, systems and policies (e520)

e 5150 **Architecture and construction services**
Services and programmes for design, construction and maintenance of residential, commercial, industrial and public buildings, such as house-building, the operationalization of design principles, building codes, regulations and standards, including those who provide these services.

e 5151 **Architecture and construction systems**
Administrative control and monitoring mechanisms that govern the planning, design, construction and maintenance of residential, commercial, industrial and public buildings, such as for implementing and monitoring building codes, construction standards, and fire and life safety standards.

e 5152 **Architecture and construction policies**
Legislation, regulations and standards that govern the planning, design, construction and maintenance of residential, commercial, industrial and public buildings, such as policies on building codes, construction standards, and fire and life safety standards.

e 5158 **Architecture and construction services, systems and policies, other specified**

e 5159 **Architecture and construction services, systems and policies, unspecified**

e 520 **Open space planning services, systems and policies**
Services, systems and policies for the planning, design, development and maintenance of public lands, (e.g. parks, forests, shorelines, wetlands) and private lands in the rural, suburban and urban context.

Exclusion: architecture and construction services, systems and policies (e515)

e 5200   Open space planning services
Services and programmes aimed at planning, creating and maintaining urban, suburban, rural, recreational, conservation and environmental space, meeting and commercial open spaces (plazas, open-air markets) and pedestrian and vehicular transportation routes for intended uses, including those who provide these services.

Exclusions: products for design, building and construction for public (e150) and private (e155) use; products of land development (e160)

e 5201   Open space planning systems
Administrative control and monitoring mechanisms, such as for the implementation of local, regional or national planning acts, design codes, heritage or conservation policies and environmental planning policy, that govern the planning, design, development and maintenance of open space, including rural, suburban and urban land, parks, conservation areas and wildlife reserves.

e 5202   Open space planning policies
Legislation, regulations and standards that govern the planning, design, development and maintenance of open space, including rural land, suburban land, urban land, parks, conservation areas and wildlife reserves, such as local, regional or national planning acts, design codes, heritage or conservation policies, and environmental planning policies.

e 5208   Open space planning services, systems and policies, other specified

e 5209   Open space planning services, systems and policies, unspecified

e 525   Housing services, systems and policies
Services, systems and policies for the provision of shelters, dwellings or lodging for people.

e 5250   Housing services
Services and programmes aimed at locating, providing and maintaining houses or shelters for persons to live in, such as estate agencies, housing organizations, shelters for homeless people, including those who provide these services.

e 5251   Housing systems
Administrative control and monitoring mechanisms that govern housing or sheltering of people, such as systems for implementing and monitoring housing policies.

e 5252   **Housing policies**
Legislation, regulations and standards that govern housing or sheltering of people, such as legislation and policies for determination of eligibility for housing or shelter, policies concerning government involvement in developing and maintaining housing, and policies concerning how and where housing is developed.

e 5258   **Housing services, systems and policies, other specified**

e 5259   **Housing services, systems and policies, unspecified**

e 530   Utilities services, systems and policies
Services, systems and policies for publicly provided utilities, such as water, fuel, electricity, sanitation, public transportation and essential services.

Exclusion: civil protection services, systems and policies (e545)

e 5300   **Utilities services**
Services and programmes supplying the population as a whole with essential energy (e.g. fuel and electricity), sanitation, water and other essential services (e.g. emergency repair services) for residential and commercial consumers, including those who provide these services.

e 5301   **Utilities systems**
Administrative control and monitoring mechanisms that govern the provision of utilities services, such as health and safety boards and consumer councils.

e 5302   **Utilities policies**
Legislation, regulations and standards that govern the provision of utilities services, such as health and safety standards governing delivery and supply of water and fuel, sanitation practices in communities, and policies for other essential services and supply during shortages or natural disasters.

e 5308   **Utilities services, systems and policies, other specified**

e 5309   **Utilities services, systems and policies, unspecified**

e 535   Communication services, systems and policies
Services, systems and policies for the transmission and exchange of information.

e 5350   **Communication services**
Services and programmes aimed at transmitting information by a variety of methods such as telephone, fax, surface and air mail, electronic mail

and other computer-based systems (e.g. telephone relay, teletype, teletext, and internet services), including those who provide these services.

Exclusion: media services (e5600)

e 5351   Communication systems
Administrative control and monitoring mechanisms, such as telecommunication regulation authorities and other such bodies, that govern the transmission of information by a variety of methods, including telephone, fax, surface and air mail, electronic mail and computer-based systems.

e 5352   Communication policies
Legislation, regulations and standards that govern the transmission of information by a variety of methods including telephone, fax, post office, electronic mail and computer-based systems, such as eligibility for access to communication services, requirements for a postal address, and standards for provision of telecommunications.

e 5358   Communication services, systems and policies, other specified

e 5359   Communication services, systems and policies, unspecified

e 540   Transportation services, systems and policies
Services, systems and policies for enabling people or goods to move or be moved from one location to another.

e 5400   Transportation services
Services and programmes aimed at moving persons or goods by road, paths, rail, air or water, by public or private transport, including those who provide these services.

Exclusion: products for personal mobility and transportation (e115)

e 5401   Transportation systems
Administrative control and monitoring mechanisms that govern the moving of persons or goods by road, paths, rail, air or water, such as systems for determining eligibility for operating vehicles and, implementation and monitoring of health and safety standards related to use of different types of transportation.

Exclusion: social security services, systems and policies (e570)

e 5402   Transportation policies
Legislation, regulations and standards that govern the moving of persons or goods by road, paths, rail, air or water, such as transportation planning

acts and policies, policies for the provision and access to public transportation.

e 5408   Transportation services, systems and policies, other specified

e 5409   Transportation services, systems and policies, unspecified

e 545   Civil protection services, systems and policies
Services, systems and policies aimed at safeguarding people and property.

Exclusion: utilities services, systems and policies (e530)

e 5450   Civil protection services
Services and programmes organized by the community and aimed at safeguarding people and property, such as fire, police, emergency and ambulance services, including those who provide these services.

e 5451   Civil protection systems
Administrative control and monitoring mechanisms that govern the safeguarding of people and property, such as systems by which provision of police, fire, emergency and ambulance services are organized.

e 5452   Civil protection policies
Legislation, regulations and standards that govern the safeguarding of people and property, such as policies governing provision of police, fire, emergency and ambulance services.

e 5458   Civil protection services, systems and policies, other specified

e 5459   Civil protection services, systems and policies, unspecified

e 550   Legal services, systems and policies
Services, systems and policies concerning the legislation and other law of a country.

e 5500   Legal services
Services and programmes aimed at providing the authority of the state as defined in law, such as courts, tribunals and other agencies for hearing and settling civil litigation and criminal trials, attorney representation, services of notaries, mediation, arbitration and correctional or penal facilities, including those who provide these services.

e 5501   Legal systems
Administrative control and monitoring mechanisms that govern the administration of justice, such as systems for implementing and

monitoring formal rules (e.g. laws, regulations, customary law, religious law, international laws and conventions).

e 5502   Legal policies
Legislation, regulations and standards, such as laws, customary law, religious law, international laws and conventions, that govern the administration of justice.

e 5508   Legal services, systems and policies, other specified

e 5509   Legal services, systems and policies, unspecified

e 555   Associations and organizational services, systems and policies
Services, systems and policies relating to groups of people who have joined together in the pursuit of common, noncommercial interests, often with an associated membership structure.

e 5550   Associations and organizational services
Services and programmes provided by people who have joined together in the pursuit of common, noncommercial interests with people who have the same interests, where the provision of such services may be tied to membership, such as associations and organizations providing recreation and leisure, sporting, cultural, religious and mutual aid services.

e 5551   Associations and organizational systems
Administrative control and monitoring mechanisms that govern the relationships and activities of people coming together with common noncommercial interests and the establishment and conduct of associations and organizations such as mutual aid organizations, recreational and leisure organizations, cultural and religious associations and not-for-profit organizations.

e 5552   Associations and organizational policies
Legislation, regulations and standards that govern the relationships and activities of people coming together with common noncommercial interests, such as policies that govern the establishment and conduct of associations and organizations, including mutual aid organizations, recreational and leisure organizations, cultural and religious associations and not-for-profit organizations.

e 5558   Associations and organizational services, systems and policies, other specified

e 5559   Associations and organizational services, systems and policies, unspecified

e 560   Media services, systems and policies
Services, systems and policies for the provision of mass communication through radio, television, newspapers and internet.

e 5600   Media services
Services and programmes aimed at providing mass communication, such as radio, television, closed captioning services, press reporting services, newspapers, Braille services and computer-based mass communication (world wide web, internet), including those who provide these services.

Exclusion: communication services (e5350)

e 5601   Media systems
Administrative control and monitoring mechanisms that govern the provision of news and information to the general public, such as standards that govern the content, distribution, dissemination, access to and methods of communicating via radio, television, press reporting services, newspapers and computer-based mass communication (world wide web, internet).

Inclusions: requirements to provide closed captions on television, Braille versions of newspapers or other publications, and teletext radio transmissions

Exclusion: communication systems (e5351)

e 5602   Media policies
Legislation, regulations and standards that govern the provision of news and information to the general public, such as policies that govern the content, distribution, dissemination, access to and methods of communicating via radio, television, press reporting services, newspapers and computer-based mass communication (world wide web, internet).

Exclusion: communication policies (e5352)

e 5608   Media services, systems and policies, other specified

e 5609   Media services, systems and policies, unspecified

e 565   Economic services, systems and policies
Services, systems and policies related to the overall system of production, distribution, consumption and use of goods and services.

Exclusion: social security services, systems and policies (e570)

e 5650   **Economic services**
Services and programmes aimed at the overall production, distribution, consumption and use of goods and services, such as the private commercial sector (e.g. businesses, corporations, private for-profit ventures), the public sector (e.g. public, commercial services such as cooperatives and corporations), financial organizations (e.g. banks and insurance services), including those who provide these services.

Exclusions: utilities services (e5300); labour and employment services (e5900)

e 5651   **Economic systems**
Administrative control and monitoring mechanisms that govern the production, distribution, consumption and use of goods and services, such as systems for implementing and monitoring economic policies.

Exclusions: utilities systems (e5301); labour and employment systems (e5901)

e 5652   **Economic policies**
Legislation, regulations and standards that govern the production, distribution, consumption and use of goods and services, such as economic doctrines adopted and implemented by governments.

Exclusions: utilities policies (e5302); labour and employment policies (e5902)

e 5658   **Economic services, systems and policies, other specified**

e 5659   **Economic services, systems and policies, unspecified**

e 570   **Social security services, systems and policies**
Services, systems and policies aimed at providing income support to people who, because of age, poverty, unemployment, health condition or disability, require public assistance that is funded either by general tax revenues or contributory schemes.

Exclusion: economic services, systems and policies (e565)

e 5700   **Social security services**
Services and programmes aimed at providing income support to people who, because of age, poverty, unemployment, health condition or disability, require public assistance that is funded either by general tax revenues or contributory schemes, such as services for determining eligibility, delivering or distributing assistance payments for the following types of programmes: social assistance programmes (e.g. non-contributory welfare, poverty or other needs-based compensation), social

insurance programmes (e.g. contributory accident or unemployment insurance), and disability and related pension schemes (e.g. income replacement), including those who provide these services.

Exclusions: health services (e5800)

e 5701 **Social security systems**
Administrative control and monitoring mechanisms that govern the programmes and schemes that provide income support to people who, because of age, poverty, unemployment, health condition or disability, require public assistance, such as systems for the implementation of rules and regulations governing the eligibility for social assistance, welfare, unemployment insurance payments, pensions and disability benefits.

e 5702 **Social security policies**
Legislation, regulations and standards that govern the programmes and schemes that provide income support to people who, because of age, poverty, unemployment, health condition or disability, require public assistance, such as legislation and regulations governing the eligibility for social assistance, welfare, unemployment insurance payments, disability and related pensions and disability benefits.

e 5708 **Social security services, systems and policies, other specified**

e 5709 **Social security services, systems and policies, unspecified**

e 575 **General social support services, systems and policies**
Services, systems and policies aimed at providing support to those requiring assistance in areas such as shopping, housework, transport, child care, respite care, self-care and care of others, in order to function more fully in society.

Exclusions: social security services, systems and policies (e570); personal care providers and personal assistants (e340); health services, systems and policies (e580)

e 5750 **General social support services**
Services and programmes aimed at providing social support to people who, because of age, poverty, unemployment, health condition or disability, require public assistance in the areas of shopping, housework, transport, self-care and care of others, in order to function more fully in society.

> **e 57500** **Informal care of child or adult by family and friends**

> **e 57501** **Family day care provided in home of service provider**

> **e 57502** **Child or adult care service centre - profit and non-profit**

e 57508   General social support services, other specified

e 57509   General social support services, unspecified

e 5751   **General social support systems**
Administrative control and monitoring mechanisms that govern the
programmes and schemes that provide social support to people who,
because of age, poverty, unemployment, health condition or disability,
require such support, including systems for the implementation of rules
and regulations governing eligibility for social support services and the
provision of these services.

e 5752   **General social support policies**
Legislation, regulations and standards that govern the programme and
schemes that provide social support to people who, because of age,
poverty, unemployment, health condition or disability, require such
support, including legislation and regulations governing eligibility for
social support.

e 5758   General social support services, systems and policies, other specified

e 5759   General social support services, systems and policies, unspecified

e 580   **Health services, systems and policies**
Services, systems and policies for preventing and treating health problems,
providing medical rehabilitation and promoting a healthy lifestyle.

Exclusion: general social support services, systems and policies (e575)

e 5800   **Health services**
Services and programmes at a local, community, regional, state or
national level, aimed at delivering interventions to individuals for their
physical, psychological and social well-being, such as health promotion
and disease prevention services, primary care services, acute care,
rehabilitation and long-term care services; services that are publicly or
privately funded, delivered on a short-term, long-term, periodic or one-
time basis, in a variety of service settings such as community, home-based,
school and work settings, general hospitals, speciality hospitals, clinics,
and residential and non-residential care facilities, including those who
provide these services.

e 5801   **Health systems**
Administrative control and monitoring mechanisms that govern the
range of services provided to individuals for their physical, psychological
and social well-being, in a variety of settings including community, home-
based, school and work settings, general hospitals, speciality hospitals,

clinics, and residential and non-residential care facilities, such as systems for implementing regulations and standards that determine eligibility for services, provision of devices, assistive technology or other adapted equipment, and legislation such as health acts that govern features of a health system such as accessibility, universality, portability, public funding and comprehensiveness.

e 5802   Health policies
Legislation, regulations and standards that govern the range of services provided to individuals for their physical, psychological and social well-being, in a variety of settings including community, home-based, school and work settings, general hospitals, speciality hospitals, clinics, and residential and non-residential care facilities, such as policies and standards that determine eligibility for services, provision of devices, assistive technology or other adapted equipment, and legislation such as health acts that govern features of a health system such as accessibility, universality, portability, public funding and comprehensiveness.

e 5808   Health services, systems and policies, other specified

e 5809   Health services, systems and policies, unspecified

e 585   Education and training services, systems and policies
Services, systems and policies for the acquisition, maintenance and improvement of knowledge, expertise and vocational or artistic skills. See UNESCO's International Standard Classification of Education (ISCED-1997).

e 5850   Education and training services
Services and programmes concerned with general education and the acquisition, maintenance and improvement of knowledge, expertise and vocational or artistic skills, such as those provided for different levels of education (e.g. preschool, primary school, secondary school, post-secondary institutions, professional programmes, training and skills programmes, apprenticeships and continuing education), including those who provide these services.

e 5851   Education and training systems
Administrative control and monitoring mechanisms that govern the delivery of education programmes, such as systems for the implementation of policies and standards that determine eligibility for public or private education and special needs-based programmes; local, regional or national boards of education or other authoritative bodies that govern features of the education systems, including curricula, size of classes, numbers of schools in a region, fees and subsidies, special meal programmes and after-school care services.

e 5852   Education and training policies
Legislation, regulations and standards that govern the delivery of
education programme, such as policies and standards that determine
eligibility for public or private education and special needs-based
programmes, and dictate the structure of local, regional or national
boards of education or other authoritative bodies that govern features of
the education system, including curricula, size of classes, numbers of
schools in a region, fees and subsidies, special meal programmes and
after-school care services.

e 5853   Special education and training services
Services and programmes concerned with special education and the
acquisition, maintenance and improvement of knowledge, expertise and
vocational or artistic skills, such as those provided for different levels of
education (e.g. preschool, primary school, secondary school, post-
secondary institutions, professional programmes, training and skills
programmes, apprenticeships and continuing education), including
those who provide these services.

e 5854   Special education and training systems
Administrative control and monitoring mechanisms that govern the
delivery of special education programmes, such as systems for the
implementation of policies and standards that determine eligibility for
public or private education and special needs-based programmes; local,
regional or national boards of education or other authoritative bodies
that govern features of the education systems, including curricula, size of
classes, numbers of schools in a region, fees and subsidies, special meal
programmes and after-school care services.

e 5855   Special education and training policies
Legislation, regulations and standards that govern the delivery of special
education programmes, such as policies and standards that determine
eligibility for public or private education and special needs-based
programmes, and dictate the structure of local, regional or national
boards of education or other authoritative bodies that govern features of
the education system, including curricula, size of classes, numbers of
schools in a region, fees and subsidies, special meal programmes and
after-school care services.

e 5858   Education and training services, systems and policies, other specified

e 5859   Education and training services, systems and policies, unspecified

e 590   Labour and employment services, systems and policies
Services, systems and policies related to finding suitable work for persons who are
unemployed or looking for different work, or to support individuals already
employed who are seeking promotion.

Exclusion: economic services, systems and policies (e565), general and specialized education services, systems and policies (e585)

e 5900   Labour and employment services
Services and programmes provided by local, regional or national governments, or private organizations to find suitable work for persons who are unemployed or looking for different work, or to support individuals already employed, such as services of employment search and preparation, reemployment, job placement, outplacement, vocational follow-up, occupational health and safety services, and work environment services (e.g. ergonomics, human resources and personnel management services, labour relations services, professional association services), including those who provide these services.

e 5901   Labour and employment systems
Administrative control and monitoring mechanisms that govern the distribution of occupations and other forms of remunerative work in the economy, such as systems for implementing policies and standards for employment creation, employment security, designated and competitive employment, labour standards and law, and trade unions.

e 5902   Labour and employment policies
Legislation, regulations and standards that govern the distribution of occupations and other forms of remunerative work in the economy, such as standards and policies for employment creation, employment security, designated and competitive employment, labour standards and law, and trade unions.

e 5908   Labour and employment services, systems and policies, other specified

e 5909   Labour and employment services, systems and policies, unspecified

e 595   **Political services, systems and policies**
Services, systems and policies related to voting, elections and governance of countries, regions and communities, as well as international organizations.

e 5950   Political services
Services and structures such as local, regional and national governments, international organizations and the people who are elected or nominated to positions within these structures, such as the United Nations, European Union, governments, regional authorities, local village authorities, traditional leaders.

e 5951   Political systems
Structures and related operations that organise political and economic power in a society, such as executive and legislative branches of

government, and the constitutional or other legal sources from which they derive their authority, such as political organizational doctrine, constitutions, agencies of executive and legislative branches of government, the military.

e 5952 **Political policy**
Laws and policies formulated and enforced through political systems that govern the operation of the political system, such as policies governing election campaigns, registration of political parties, voting, and members in international political organizations, including treaties, constitutional and other law governing legislation and regulation.

e 5958 **Political services, systems and policies, other specified**

e 5959 **Political services, systems and policies, unspecified**

e 598 Services, systems and policies, other specified

e 599 Services, systems and policies, unspecified

ICF

Annexes

Annex 1

Taxonomic and terminological issues

The ICF classification is organized in a hierarchical scheme keeping in mind the following standard taxonomic principles:

- The components of Body Functions and Structures, Activities and Participation, and Environmental Factors are classified independently. Hence, a term included under one component is not repeated under another.

- Within each component, the categories are arranged in a stem–branch–leaf scheme, so that a lower-level category shares the attributes of the higher-level categories of which it is a member.

- Categories are mutually exclusive, i.e. no two categories at the same level share exactly the same attributes. However, this should not be confused with the use of more than one category to classify a particular individual's functioning. Such a practice is allowed, indeed encouraged, where necessary.

1. Terms for categories in ICF

Terms are the designation of defined concepts in linguistic expressions, such as words or phrases. Most of the terms over which confusion arises are used with common-sense meanings in everyday speech and writing. For example, impairment, disability and handicap are often used interchangeably in everyday contexts, although in the 1980 version of ICIDH these terms had stipulated definitions, which gave them a precisely defined meaning. During the revision process, the term "handicap" was abandoned and "disability" was used as an umbrella term for all three perspectives – body, individual and societal. Clarity and precision, however, are needed to define the various concepts, so that appropriate terms may be chosen to express each of the underlying concepts unambiguously. This is particularly important because ICF, as a written classification, will be translated into many languages. Beyond a common understanding of the concepts, it is also essential that an agreement be reached on the term that best reflects the content in each language. There may be many alternatives, and decisions should be made based on accuracy, acceptability, and overall usefulness. It is hoped that the usefulness of ICF will go in parallel with its clarity.

With this aim in mind, notes on some of the terms used in ICF follow:

Well-being is a general term encompassing the total universe of human life domains, including physical, mental and social aspects, that make up what can be called a "good life". Health domains are a subset of domains that make up the total universe of human life. This relationship is presented in Fig. 1.

Health states and health domains: A health state is the level of functioning within a given health domain of ICF. Health domains denote areas of life that are interpreted to be within the "health" notion, such as those which, for health systems purposes, can be defined as the primary responsibility of the health system. ICF does not dictate a fixed boundary between health and health-related domains. There may be a grey zone depending on differing

Fig. 1 The universe of well-being

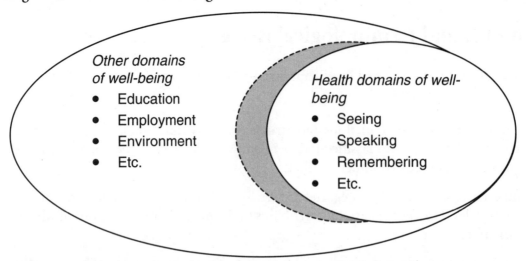

conceptualizations of health and health-related elements which can then be mapped onto the ICF domains.

Health-related states and health-related domains: A health-related state is the level of functioning within a given health-related domain of ICF. Health-related domains are those areas of functioning that, while they have a strong relationship to a health condition, are not likely to be the primary responsibility of the health system, but rather of other systems contributing to overall well-being. In ICF, only those domains of well-being related to health are covered.

Health condition is an umbrella term for disease (acute or chronic), disorder, injury or trauma. A health condition may also include other circumstances such as pregnancy, ageing, stress, congenital anomaly, or genetic predisposition. Health conditions are coded using ICD-10.

Functioning is an umbrella term for body functions, body structures, activities and participation. It denotes the positive aspects of the interaction between an individual (with a health condition) and that individual's contextual factors (environmental and personal factors).

Disability is an umbrella term for impairments, activity limitations and participation restrictions. It denotes the negative aspects of the interaction between an individual (with a health condition) and that individual's contextual factors (environmental and personal factors).

Body functions are the physiological functions of body systems, including psychological functions. "Body" refers to the human organism as a whole, and thus includes the brain. Hence, mental (or psychological) functions are subsumed under body functions. The standard for these functions is considered to be the statistical norm for humans.

Body structures are the structural or anatomical parts of the body such as organs, limbs and their components classified according to body systems. The standard for these structures is considered to be the statistical norm for humans.

Impairment is a loss or abnormality in body structure or physiological function (including mental functions). Abnormality here is used strictly to refer to a significant variation from established statistical norms (i.e. as a deviation from a population mean within measured standard norms) and should be used only in this sense.

Activity is the execution of a task or action by an individual. It represents the individual perspective of functioning.

Activity limitations[24] are difficulties an individual may have in executing activities. An activity limitation may range from a slight to a severe deviation in terms of quality or quantity in executing the activity in a manner or to the extent that is expected of people without the health condition.

Participation is a person's involvement in a life situation. It represents the societal perspective of functioning.

Participation restrictions[25] are problems an individual may experience in involvement in life situations. The presence of a participation restriction is determined by comparing an individual's participation to that which is expected of an individual without disability in that culture or society.

Contextual factors are the factors that together constitute the complete context of an individual's life, and, in particular, the background against which health states are classified in ICF. There are two components of contextual factors: Environmental Factors and Personal Factors.

Environmental factors constitute a component of ICF, and refer to all aspects of the external or extrinsic world that form the context of an individual's life and, as such, have an impact on that person's functioning. Environmental factors include the physical world and its features, the human-made physical world, other people in different relationships and roles, attitudes and values, social systems and services, and policies, rules and laws.

Personal factors are contextual factors that relate to the individual, such as age, gender, social status, life experiences and so on, which are not currently classified in ICF but which users may incorporate in their applications of the classification.

Facilitators are factors in a person's environment that, through their absence or presence, improve functioning and reduce disability. These include aspects such as a physical environment that is accessible, the availability of relevant assistive technology, and positive attitudes of people towards disability, as well as services, systems and policies that aim to increase the involvement of all people with a health condition in all areas of life. Absence of a factor can also be facilitating, for example the absence of stigma or negative attitudes. Facilitators can prevent an impairment or activity limitation from becoming a participation restriction, since the actual performance of an action is enhanced, despite the person's problem with capacity.

---

[24] "Activity limitation" replaces the term "disability" used in the 1980 version of ICIDH.

[25] "Participation restriction" replaces the term "handicap" used in the 1980 version of ICIDH.

Barriers are factors in a person's environment that, through their absence or presence, limit functioning and create disability. These include aspects such as a physical environment that is inaccessible, lack of relevant assistive technology, and negative attitudes of people towards disability, as well as services, systems and policies that are either nonexistent or that hinder the involvement of all people with a health condition in all areas of life.

Capacity is a construct that indicates, as a qualifier, the highest probable level of functioning that a person may reach in a domain in the Activities and Participation list at a given moment. Capacity is measured in a uniform or standard environment, and thus reflects the environmentally adjusted ability of the individual. The Environmental Factors component can be used to describe the features of this uniform or standard environment.

Performance is a construct that describes, as a qualifier, what individuals do in their current environment, and so brings in the aspect of a person's involvement in life situations. The current environment is also described using the Environmental Factors component.

2. ICF as a classification

In order to understand the overall classification of ICF, it is important to understand its structure. This is reflected in the definitions of the following terms and illustrated in Fig. 2.

Classification is the overall structure and universe of ICF. In the hierarchy, this is the top term.

Parts of the classification are each of the two main subdivisions of the classification.

- Part 1 covers Functioning and Disability
- Part 2 covers Contextual Factors

Components are each of the two main subdivisions of the parts.

The components of Part 1 are:

- Body Functions and Structures
- Activities and Participation.

The components of Part 2 are:

- Environmental Factors
- Personal Factors (not classified in ICF).

Constructs are defined through the use of qualifiers with relevant codes.

There are four constructs for Part 1 and one for Part 2.

Fig. 2 Structure of ICF

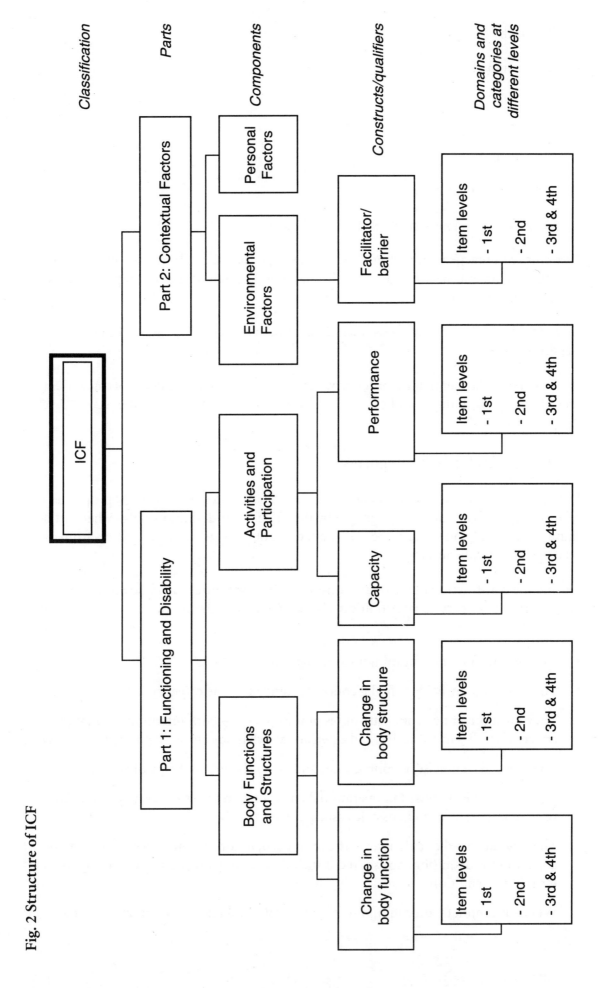

For Part 1, the constructs are:

- change in body function

- change in body structure

- capacity

- performance.

For Part 2, the construct is:

- facilitators or barriers in environmental factors.

Domains are a practical, meaningful set of related physiological functions, anatomical structures, actions, tasks, or areas of life. Domains make up the different chapters and blocks within each component.

Categories are classes and subclasses within a domain of a component, i.e. units of classification.

Levels make up the hierarchical order providing indications as to the detail of categories (i.e. granularity of the domains and categories). The first level comprises all the second-level items, and so on.

3. Definitions for ICF categories

Definitions are statements that set out the essential attributes (i.e. qualities, properties or relationships) of the concept designated by the category. A definition states what sort of thing or phenomenon the term denotes and, operationally, notes how it differs from other related things or phenomena.

During the construction of the definitions of the ICF categories, the following ideal characteristics of operational definitions, including inclusions and exclusions, were kept in mind.

- Definitions should be meaningful and logically consistent.

- They must uniquely identify the concept intended by the category.

- They must present essential attributes of the concept – both intentional (what the concept signifies intrinsically) and extensional (what objects or phenomena it refers to).

- They should be precise, unambiguous, and cover the full meaning of the term.

- They should be expressed in operational terms (e.g. in terms of severity, duration, relative importance, and possible associations).

- They should avoid circularity, i.e. the term itself, or any synonym for it, should not appear in the definition, nor should it include a term defined elsewhere using the first term in its definition.

- Where appropriate, they should refer to possible etiological or interactive factors.

- They must fit the attributes of the higher-ranking terms (e.g. a third-level term should include the general characteristics of the second-level category to which it belongs).

- They must be consistent with the attributes of the subordinate terms (e.g. the attributes of a second-level term cannot contradict those of third-level terms under it).

- They must not be figurative or metaphorical, but operational.

- They should make empirical statements that are observable, testable or inferable by indirect means.

- They should be expressed in neutral terms as far as possible, without undue negative connotation.

- They should be short and avoid technical terms where possible (with the exception of some Body Functions and Structures terms).

- They should have inclusions that provide synonyms and examples that take into account cultural variation and differences across the life span.

- They should have exclusions to alert users to possible confusion with related terms.

4. Additional note on terminology

Underlying the terminology of any classification is the fundamental distinction between the phenomena being classified and the structure of the classification itself. As a general matter, it is important to distinguish between the world and the terms we use to describe the world. For example, the terms 'dimension' or 'domain' could be precisely defined to refer to the world and 'component' and 'category' defined to refer only to the classification.

At the same time, there is a correspondence (i.e. a matching function) between these terms and it is possible that a wide variety of users may use these terms interchangeably. For more highly specialized requirements, for database construction and research modelling for example, it is essential for users to identify separately, and with a clearly distinct terminology, the elements of the conceptual model and those of the classification structure. Yet, it has been felt that the precision and purity that such an approach provides is not worth the price paid in a level of abstraction that might undermine the usefulness of the ICF, or more importantly to restrict the range of potential users of this classification.

Annex 2

Guidelines for coding ICF

ICF is intended for the coding of different health and health-related states.[26] Users are strongly recommended to read through the Introduction to ICF before studying the coding rules and guidelines. Furthermore, it is highly recommended that users obtain training in the use of the classification through WHO and its network of collaborating centres.

The following are features of the classification that have a bearing on its use.

1. Organization and structure

Parts of the Classification

ICF is organized into two parts.

Part 1 is composed of the following components:

- Body Functions and Body Structures

- Activities and Participation.

Part 2 is composed of the following components:

- Environmental Factors

- Personal Factors (currently not classified in the ICF).

These components are denoted by prefixes in each code:

- *b* for Body Functions and

- *s* for Body Structures

- *d* for Activities and Participation

- *e* for Environmental Factors.

The prefix *d* denotes the domains within the component of Activities and Participation. At the user's discretion, the prefix *d* can be replaced by *a* or *p*, to denote activities and participation respectively.

---

[26] The disease itself should not be coded. This can be done using the International Statistical Classification of Diseases and Related Health Problems, Tenth Revision (ICD-10), which is a classification designed to permit the systematic recording, analysis, interpretation and comparison of mortality and morbidity data on diagnoses of diseases and other health problems. Users of ICF are encouraged to use this classification in conjunction with ICD-10 (see page 4 of Introduction regarding overlap between the classifications)

The letters *b*, *s*, *d* and *e* are followed by a numeric code that starts with the chapter number (one digit), followed by the second level (two digits), and the third and fourth level[27] (one digit each). For example, in the Body Functions classification there are these codes:

b2	Sensory functions and pain	(first-level item)
b210	Seeing functions	(second-level item)
b2102	Quality of vision	(third-level item)
b21022	Contrast sensitivity	(fourth-level item)

Depending on the user's needs, any number of applicable codes can be employed at each level. To describe an individual's situation, more than one code at each level may be applicable. These may be independent or interrelated.

In ICF, a person's health state may be assigned an array of codes across the domains of the components of the classification. The maximum number of codes available for each application is 34 at the chapter level (8 body functions, 8 body structures, 9 performance and 9 capacity codes), and 362 at the second level. At the third and fourth levels, there are up to 1424 codes available, which together constitute the full version of the classification. In real-life applications of ICF, a set of 3 to 18 codes may be adequate to describe a case with two-level (three-digit) precision. Generally, the more detailed four-level version is intended for specialist services (e.g. rehabilitation outcomes, geriatrics, or mental health), whereas the two-level classification can be used for surveys and health outcome evaluation.

The domains should be coded as applicable to a given moment (i.e. as a snapshot description of an encounter), which is the default position. Use over time, however, is also possible in order to describe a trajectory over time or a process. Users should then identify their coding style and the time-frame that they use.

Chapters

Each component of the classification is organized into chapter and domain headings under which are common categories or specific items. For example, in the Body Functions classification, Chapter 1 deals with all mental functions.

Blocks

The chapters are often subdivided into "blocks" of categories. For example, in Chapter 3 of the Activities and Participation classification (Communication), there are three blocks: Communicating—Receiving (d310–d329), Communicating—Producing (d330–d349), and Conversation and using communication devices and techniques (d350– d369). Blocks are provided as a convenience to the user and, strictly speaking, are not part of the structure of the classification and normally will not be used for coding purposes.

---

[27] Only the Body Functions and Body Structure classifications contain fourth-level items.

Categories

Within each chapter there are individual two-, three- or four-level categories, each with a short definition and inclusions and exclusions as appropriate to assist in the selection of the appropriate code.

Definitions

ICF gives operational definitions of the health and health-related categories, as opposed to "vernacular" or layperson's definitions. These definitions describe the essential attributes of each domain (e.g. qualities, properties, and relationships) and contain information as to what is included and excluded in each category. The definitions also contain commonly used anchor points for assessment, for application in surveys and questionnaires, or alternatively, for the results of assessment instruments coded in ICF terms. For example, visual acuity functions are defined in terms of monocular and binocular acuity at near and far distances so that the severity of visual acuity difficulty can be coded as none, mild, moderate, severe or total.

Inclusion terms

Inclusion terms are listed after the definition of many categories. They are provided as a guide to the content of the category, and are not meant to be exhaustive. In the case of second-level items, the inclusions cover all embedded, third-level items.

Exclusion terms

Exclusion terms are provided where, owing to the similarity with another term, application might prove difficult. For example, it might be thought that the category "Toileting" includes the category "Caring for body parts". To distinguish the two, however, "Toileting" is excluded from category d520 "Caring for body parts" and coded to d530.

Other specified

At the end of each embedded set of third- or fourth-level items, and at the end of each chapter, are "other specified" categories (uniquely identified by the final code number 8). These allow for the coding of aspects of functioning that are not included within any of the other specific categories. When "other specified" is employed, the user should specify the new item in an additional list.

Unspecified

The last categories within each embedded set of third- or fourth-level items, and at the end of each chapter, are "unspecified" categories that allow for the coding of functions that fit within the group but for which there is insufficient information to permit the assignment of a more specific category. This code has the same meaning as the second- or third-level term immediately above, without any additional information (for blocks, the "other specified" and "unspecified" categories are joined into a single item, but are always identified by the final code number 9).

Qualifiers

The ICF codes require the use of one or more qualifiers, which denote, for example, the magnitude of the level of health or severity of the problem at issue. Qualifiers are coded as one, two or more numbers after a point. Use of any code should be accompanied by at least one qualifier. Without qualifiers codes have no inherent meaning (by default, WHO interprets incomplete codes as signifying the absence of a problem -- xxx.00).

The first qualifier for Body Functions and Structures, the performance and capacity qualifiers for Activities and Participation, and the first qualifier for Environmental Factors all describe the extent of problems in the respective component.

All components are quantified using the same generic scale. Having a problem may mean an impairment, limitation, restriction or barrier, depending on the construct. Appropriate qualifying words as shown in brackets below should be chosen according to the relevant classification domain (where xxx stands for the second-level domain number):

xxx.0	NO problem	(none, absent, negligible,…)	0–4 %
xxx.1	MILD problem	(slight, low,…)	5–24 %
xxx.2	MODERATE problem	(medium, fair,…)	25–49 %
xxx.3	SEVERE problem	(high, extreme,…)	50–95 %
xxx.4	COMPLETE problem	(total,…)	96–100 %
xxx.8	not specified		
xxx.9	not applicable		

Broad ranges of percentages are provided for those cases in which calibrated assessment instruments or other standards are available to quantify the impairment, capacity limitation, performance problem or environmental barrier/facilitator. For example, when "no problem" or "complete problem" is coded, this may have a margin of error of up to 5%. A "moderate problem" is defined as up to half of the scale of total difficulty. The percentages are to be calibrated in different domains with reference to population standards as percentiles. For this quantification to be used in a universal manner, assessment procedures have to be developed through research.

In the case of the Environmental Factors component, this first qualifier can also be used to denote the extent of positive aspects of the environment, or facilitators. To denote facilitators, the same 0–4 scale can be used, but the point is replaced by a plus sign: e.g. e110+2. Environmental factors can be coded either (i) in relation to each component; or (ii) without relation to each component (see section 3 below). The first style is preferable since it identifies the impact and attribution more clearly.

Additional qualifiers

For different users, it might be appropriate and helpful to add other kinds of information to the coding of each item. There are a variety of additional qualifiers that could be useful, as mentioned later.

Coding positive aspects

At the user's discretion coding scales can be developed to capture the positive aspects of functioning:

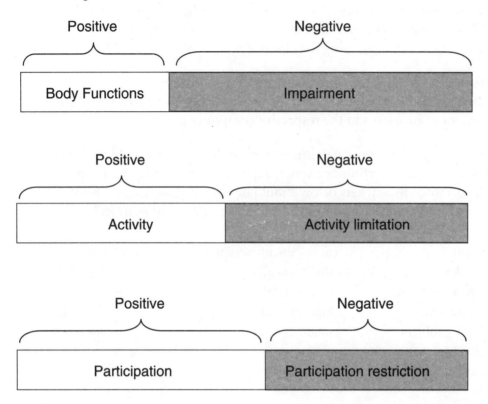

2. General coding rules

The following rules are essential for accurate retrieval of information for the various uses of the classification.

Select an array of codes to form an individual's profile

ICF classifies health and health-related states and therefore requires the assigning of a series of codes that best describe the profile of the person's functioning. ICF is not an "event classification" like ICD-10 in which a particular health condition is classified with a single code. As the functioning of a person can be affected at the body, individual and societal level, the user should always take into consideration all components of the classification, namely Body Functions and Structures, Activities and Participation, and Environmental Factors. Though it is impractical to expect that all the possible codes will be used for every encounter, depending on the setting of the encounter users will select the most salient codes for their purpose to describe a given health experience.

Code relevant information

Coded information is always in the context of a health condition. Although to use the codes it is not necessary to trace the links between the health condition and the aspects of functioning and disability that are coded, ICF is a health classification and so presumes the presence of a health condition of some kind. Therefore, information about what a person does or does not choose to do is not related to a functioning problem associated with a health condition and should not be coded. For example, if a person decides not to begin new relationships with his or her neighbours for reasons other than health, then it is not appropriate to use category d7200, which includes the actions of forming relationships. Conversely, if the person's decision is linked to a health condition (e.g. depression), then the code should be applied.

Information that reflects the person's feeling of involvement or satisfaction with the level of functioning is currently not coded in ICF. Further research may provide additional qualifiers that will allow this information to be coded.

Only those aspects of the person's functioning relevant to a predefined time-frame should be coded. Functions that relate to an earlier encounter and have no bearing on the current encounter should not be recorded.

Code explicit information

When assigning codes, the user should not make an inference about the inter-relationship between an impairment of body functions or structure, activity limitation or participation restriction. For example, if a person has a limitation in functioning in moving around, it is not justifiable to assume that the person has an impairment of movement functions. Similarly, from the fact that a person has a limited capacity to move around it is unwarranted to infer that he or she has a performance problem in moving around. The user must obtain explicit information on Body Functions and Structures and on capacity and performance separately (in some instances, mental functions for example, an inference from other observations is required since the body function in question is not directly observable).

Code specific information

Health and health-related states should be recorded as specifically as possible, by assigning the most appropriate ICF category. For example, the most specific code for a person with night blindness is b21020 "Light sensitivity". If, however, for some reason this level of detail cannot be applied, the corresponding "parent" code in the hierarchy can be used instead (in this case, b2102 Quality of vision, b210 Seeing functions, or b2 Sensory functions and pain).

To identify the appropriate code easily and quickly, the use of the ICF Browser,[28] which provides a search engine function with an electronic index of the full version of the classification, is strongly recommended. Alternatively, the alphabetical index can be used.

3. Coding conventions for the Environmental Factors component

For the coding of environmental factors, three coding conventions are open for use:

Convention 1

Environmental factors are coded alone, without relating these codes to body functions, body structures or activities and participation.

---

[28] The ICF Browser in different languages can be downloaded from the ICF website: http://www.who.int/classifications/icf

Body functions   _____
Body structures   _____
Activities and Participation _____
Environment   _____

Convention 2

Environmental factors are coded for every component.

Body functions   _____ E code _____
Body structures   _____ E code _____
Activities and Participation _____ E code _____

Convention 3

Environmental factors are coded for capacity and performance qualifiers in the Activities and Participation component for every item.

Performance qualifier _____ E code _____
Capacity qualifier   _____ E code _____

4. Component-specific coding rules

4.1 *Coding body functions*

Definitions

Body functions are the physiological functions of body systems (including psychological functions). *Impairments* are problems in body function or structure as a significant deviation or loss.

Using the qualifier for body functions

Body functions are coded with one qualifier that indicates the extent or magnitude of the impairment. The presence of an impairment can be identified as a loss or lack, reduction, addition or excess, or deviation.

The impairment of a person with hemiparesis can be described with code b7302 Power of muscles of one side of the body:

Extent of impairment (first qualifier)

b7302.__

Once an impairment is present, it can be scaled in severity using the generic qualifier. For example:

b7302.1 MILD impairment of power of muscles of one side of body   (5–24 %)
b7302.2 MODERATE impairment of power of muscles of one side of body (25–49 %)
b7302.3 SEVERE impairment of power of muscles of one side of body   (50–95 %)
b7302.4 COMPLETE impairment of power of muscles of one side of body (96–100 %)

The absence of an impairment (according to a predefined threshold level) is indicated by the value "0" for the generic qualifier. For example:

   b7302.0 NO impairment in power of muscles of one side of body

If there is insufficient information to specify the severity of the impairment, the value "8" should be used. For example, if a person's health record states that the person is suffering from weakness of the right side of the body without giving further details, then the following code can be applied:

   b7302.8 Impairment of power of muscles of one side of body, not specified

There may be situations where it is inappropriate to apply a particular code. For example, the code b650 Menstruation functions is not applicable for women before or beyond a certain age (pre-menarche or post-menopause). For these cases, the value "9" is assigned:

   b650.9 Menstruation functions, not applicable

Structural correlates of body functions

The classifications of Body Functions and Body Structures are designed to be parallel. When a body function code is used, the user should check whether the corresponding body structure code is applicable. For example, body functions include basic human senses such as b210-b229 Seeing and related functions," and their structural correlates occur between s210 and s230 as "eye and related structures".

Interrelationship between impairments

Impairments may result in other impairments; for example, muscle power may impair movement functions, heart functions may relate to respiratory functions, perception may relate to thought functions.

Identifying impairments in body functions

For those impairments that cannot always be observed directly (e.g. mental functions), the user can infer the impairment from observation of behaviour. For example, in a clinical setting memory may be assessed through standardized tests, and although it is not possible to actually "observe" brain function, depending on the results of these tests it may be reasonable to assume that the mental functions of memory are impaired.

4.2 *Coding body structures*

Definitions

Body structures are anatomical parts of the body such as organs, limbs and their components. *Impairments* are problems in body function or structure as a significant deviation or loss.

Using qualifiers for coding body structures

Body structures are coded with three qualifiers. The first qualifier describes the extent or magnitude of the impairment, the second qualifier is used to indicate the nature of the change, and the third qualifier denotes the location of the impairment.

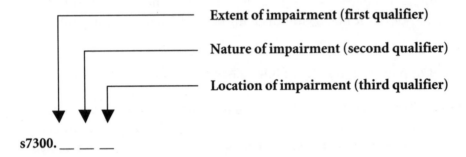

Extent of impairment (first qualifier)

Nature of impairment (second qualifier)

Location of impairment (third qualifier)

s7300. __ __ __

The descriptive schemes used for the three qualifiers are listed in Table 1.

Table 1. Scaling of qualifiers for body structures

First qualifier Extent of impairment	Second qualifier Nature of impairment	Third qualifier (suggested) Location of impairment
0 NO impairment 1 MILD impairment 2 MODERATE impairment 3 SEVERE impairment 4 COMPLETE impairment 8 not specified 9 not applicable	0 no change in structure 1 total absence 2 partial absence 3 additional part 4 aberrant dimensions 5 discontinuity 6 deviating position 7 qualitative changes in structure, including accumulation of fluid 8 not specified 9 not applicable	0 more than one region 1 right 2 left 3 both sides 4 front 5 back 6 proximal 7 distal 8 not specified 9 not applicable

4.3 *Coding the Activities and Participation component*

Definitions

Activity is the execution of a task or action by an individual. *Participation* is involvement in a life situation. *Activity limitations* are difficulties an individual may have in executing activities. *Participation restrictions* are problems an individual may experience in involvement in life situations.

The Activities and Participation classification is a single list of domains.

Using the capacity and performance qualifiers

Activities and Participation is coded with two qualifiers: the *performance* qualifier, which occupies the first digit position after the point, and the *capacity* qualifier, which occupies the second digit position after the point. The code that identifies the category from the Activities and Participation list and the two qualifiers form the default information matrix.

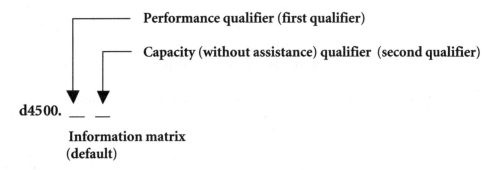

Performance qualifier (first qualifier)

Capacity (without assistance) qualifier (second qualifier)

d4500. __ __

**Information matrix
(default)**

The performance qualifier describes what an individual does in his or her current environment. Because the current environment brings in a societal context, performance as recorded by this qualifier can also be understood as "involvement in a life situation" or "the lived experience" of people in the actual context in which they live. This context includes the environmental factors – i.e. all aspects of the physical, social and attitudinal world. This features of the current environment can be coded using the Environmental Factors classification.

The capacity qualifier describes an individual's ability to execute a task or an action. This construct aims to indicate the highest probable level of functioning that a person may reach in a given domain at a given moment. To assess the full ability of the individual, one would need to have a "standardized" environment to neutralize the varying impact of different environments on the ability of the individual. This standardized environment may be: (a) an actual environment commonly used for capacity assessment in test settings; (b) in cases where this is not possible, an assumed environment which can be thought to have an uniform impact. This environment can be called the "uniform" or "standard" environment. Thus, the capacity construct reflects the environmentally adjusted ability of the individual. This adjustment has to be the same for all persons in all countries to allow international comparisons. To be precise, the features of the uniform or standard environment can be coded using the Environmental Factors component. The gap between capacity and performance reflects the difference between the impacts of the current and uniform environments and thus provides a useful guide as to what can be done to the environment of the individual to improve performance.

Typically, the capacity qualifier without assistance is used in order to describe the individual's true ability which is not enhanced by an assistance device or personal assistance. Since the performance qualifier addresses the individual's current environment, the presence of assistive devices or personal assistance or barriers can be directly observed. The nature of the facilitator or barrier can be described using the Environmental Factors classification.

Optional qualifiers

The third and fourth (optional) qualifiers provide users with the possibility of coding capacity with assistance and performance without assistance.

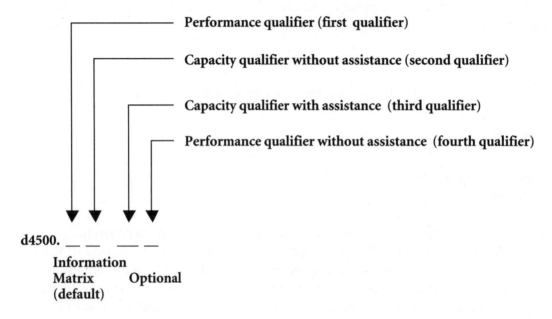

d4500. _ _   _ _

Information Matrix (default)   **Optional**

Additional qualifiers

The fifth digit position is reserved for qualifiers that may be developed in the future, such as a qualifier for involvement or subjective satisfaction.

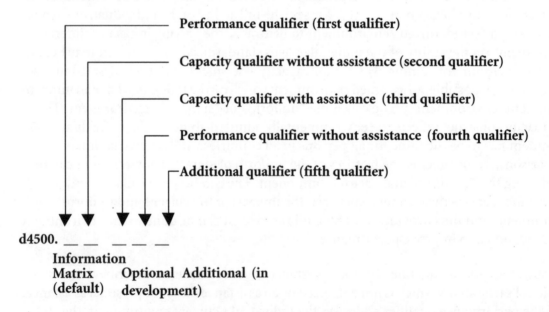

d4500. _ _   _ _ _

Information Matrix (default)   **Optional Additional (in development)**

Both capacity and performance qualifiers can further be used both with and without assistive devices or personal assistance, and in accordance with the following scale (where xxx stands for the second-level domain number):

xxx.0   NO difficulty
xxx.1   MILD difficulty

xxx.2	MODERATE difficulty
xxx.3	SEVERE difficulty
xxx.4	COMPLETE difficulty
xxx.8	not specified
xxx.9	not applicable

When to use the performance qualifier and the capacity qualifier

Either qualifier may be used for each of the categories listed. But the information conveyed in each case is different. When both qualifiers are used, the result is an aggregation of two constructs, i.e.:

d4500. 2 1 ⟶ **d4500. 2 _**

d4500._ 1

If only one qualifier is used, then the unused space should not be filled with .8 or .9, but left blank, since both of these are true assessment values and would imply that the qualifier is being used.

Examples of the application of the two qualifiers

d4500 Walking short distances

For the *performance qualifier*, this domain refers to getting around on foot, in the person's current environment, such as on different surfaces and conditions, with the use of a cane, walker, or other assistive technology, for distances less than 1 km. For example, the performance of a person who lost his leg in a work-related accident and since then has used a cane but faces moderate difficulties in walking around because the sidewalks in the neighbourhood are very steep and have a very slippery surface can be coded:

d4500.3 _ moderate restriction in performance of walking short distances

For the *capacity qualifier*, this domain refers to the an individual's ability to walk around without assistance. In order to neutralize the varying impact of different environments, the ability may be assessed in a "standardized" environment. This standardized environment may be: (a) an actual environment commonly used for capacity assessment in test settings; or (b) in cases where this is not possible, an assumed environment which can be thought to have an uniform impact. For example, the true ability of the above-mentioned person to walk without a cane in a standardized environment (such as one with flat and non-slippery surfaces) will be very limited. Therefore the person's capacity may be coded as follows:

d4500._ 3 severe capacity limitation in walking short distances

Users who wish to specify the current or standardized environment while using the performance or capacity qualifier should use the Environmental Factors classification (see coding convention 3 for Environmental Factors in section 3 above).

4.4   *Coding environmental factors*

Definitions

Environmental Factors make up the physical, social and attitudinal environment in which people live and conduct their lives.

Use of Environmental Factors

Environmental Factors is a component of Part 2 (Contextual Factors) of the classification. Environmental factors must be considered for each component of functioning and coded according to one of the three conventions described in section 3 above.

Environmental factors are to be coded from the perspective of the person whose situation is being described. For example, kerb cuts without textured paving may be coded as a facilitator for a wheelchair user but as a barrier for a blind person.

The qualifier indicates the extent to which a factor is a facilitator or a barrier. There are several reasons why an environmental factor may be a facilitator or a barrier, and to what extent. For facilitators, the coder should keep in mind issues such as the accessibility of a resource, and whether access is dependable or variable, of good or poor quality and so on. In the case of barriers, it might be relevant how often a factor hinders the person, whether the hindrance is great or small, or avoidable or not. It should also be kept in mind that an environmental factor can be a barrier either because of its presence (for example, negative attitudes towards people with disabilities) or its absence (for example, the unavailability of a needed service). The effects that environmental factors have on the lives of people with health conditions are varied and complex, and it is hoped that future research will lead to a better understanding of this interaction and, possibly, show the usefulness of a second qualifier for these factors.

In some instances, a diverse collection of environmental factors is summarized with a single term, such as poverty, development, rural or urban setting, or social capital. These summary terms are not themselves found in the classification. Rather, the coder should separate the constituent factors and code these. Once again, further research is required to determine whether there are clear and consistent sets of environmental factors that make up each of these summary terms.

First qualifier

The following is the negative and positive scale that denotes the extent to which an environmental factor acts as a barrier or a facilitator. Using a point alone denotes a barrier, whereas using the + sign instead denotes a facilitator, as indicated below:

xxx.0	NO barrier		xxx+0	NO facilitator
			xxx+1	MILD facilitator
xxx.1	MILD barrier		xxx+2	MODERATE facilitator
xxx.2	MODERATE barrier		xxx+3	SUBSTANTIAL facilitator
xxx.3	SEVERE barrier		xxx+4	COMPLETE facilitator
xxx.4	COMPLETE barrier			
			xxx+8	facilitator, not specified
xxx.8	barrier, not specified		xxx.9	not applicable
xxx.9	not applicable			

Annex 3

Possible uses of the Activities and Participation list

The Activities and Participation component is a neutral list of domains indicating various actions and life areas. Each domain contains categories at different levels ordered from general to detailed (e.g. the domain of Chapter 4 Mobility, contains categories such as d450 Walking and under it the more specific item, d4500 Walking short distances.) The list of activity and participation domains covers the full range of functioning, which can be coded at both the individual and societal levels.

As indicated in the Introduction, this list can be used in different ways to indicate the specific notions of "Activities" and "Participation", which are defined in ICF as follows:

In the context of health:

Activity is the execution of a task or action by an individual.

Participation is involvement in a life situation.

There are four alternative options for structuring the relationship between activities (a) and participation (p) in terms of the domain list:

(1) Distinct sets of ativities domains and participation domains (no overlap)

A certain set of categories is coded only as activities (i.e. tasks or actions that an individual does) and another set only as participation (i.e. involvement in life situations). The two sets, therefore, are mutually exclusive.

In this option, the sets of activity categories and participation categories is determined by the user. Each category is either an activity or a participation item, but not both. For example, the domains may be divided as follows:

a1 Learning and applying knowledge
a2 General tasks and demands
a3 Communication
a4 Mobility

p5 Self-care
p6 Domestic life
p7 Interpersonal interactions
p8 Major life areas
p9 Community, social and civic life

Coding for this structure

a *category code.* q_p q_c (a category deemed an activities item)
p *category code.* q_p q_c (a category deemed a participation item)

Where q_p = the performance qualifier and q_c = the capacity qualifier. If the performance qualifier is used, the category, whether denoted as an activities or a participation item, is interpreted in terms of the performance construct; if the capacity qualifier is used, a capacity construct is used to interpret the category, again whether denoted as an activities or a participation item.

In this way option (1) provides the full information matrix without any redundancy or overlap.

(2)   Partial overlap between sets of activities and participation domains

In this alternative, a set of categories may be interpreted as both activities and participation items; that is, the same category is thought to be open to an individual (i.e. as a task or action that an individual does) and a societal (i.e. involvement in a life situation) interpretation.

For example:

a1 Learning and applying knowledge	
a2 General tasks and demands	
a3 Communication	p3 Communication
a4 Mobility	p4 Mobility
a5 Self-care	p5 Self-care
a6 Domestic life	p6 Domestic life
	p7 Interpersonal interactions
	p8 Major life areas
	p9 Community, social and civic life

Coding for this structure

There is a restriction on how categories can be coded for this structure. It cannot be possible for a category within the "overlap" to have different values for the same qualifier (either the first qualifier for performance or the second qualifier for capacity), e.g.:

a *category*. 1 _   or   a *category*. _ 1
p *category*. 2   p *category*. _ 2

A user who chooses this option believes that codes in the overlapping categories may mean different things when they are coded in activities and not in participation, and vice versa. However, one single code has to be entered into the information matrix for the specified qualifier column.

(3)   Detailed categories as activities and broad categories as participation, with or without overlap

Another approach to applying activities and participation definitions to the domains restricts participation to the more general or broader categories within a domain (e.g. first-level categories such as chapter headings) and deems the more detailed categories to be activities (e.g. third- or fourth-level categories). This approach separates categories within some or all domains in terms of the broad versus detailed distinction. The user may deem some domains to be entirely (i.e. at all levels of detail) activities or entirely participation.

For example, d4550 Crawling may be construed as an activity while d455 Moving around may be construed as participation.

There are two possible ways of handling this approach: (a) there is no "overlap", i.e. if an item is an activity it is not participation; or (b) there may be an overlap, since some users may use the whole list for activities and only broad titles for participation.

Coding for this structure

Similar to option (1) or option (2).

(4) Use of the same domains for both activities and participation with total overlap of domains

In this option, all domains in the Activities and Participation list can be viewed as both activities and participation. Every category can be interpreted as individual functioning (activity) as well as societal functioning (participation).

For example, d330 Speaking can be seen both as an activity and as participation. A person with missing vocal cords can speak with the use of an assistive device. According to the assessments using capacity and performance qualifiers, this person has:

First qualifier
Moderate difficulty in performance (perhaps because of contextual factors such as →2 personal stress or other peoples', attitudes)

Second qualifier
Severe difficulty in capacity without assistive device →3

Third qualifier
Mild difficulty in capacity with assistive device →1

According to the ICF information matrix this person's situation should be coded as:

d330.231

According to option (4) this can also be coded as:

a330.231
p330.2

In option (4), when both performance and capacity qualifiers are used, there are two values for the same cell in the ICF information matrix: one for activities and one for participation. If these values are the same, then there is no conflict, only redundancy. However, in the case of differing values, users must develop a decision rule to code for the information matrix, since the official WHO coding style is this:

d *category* q$_p$ q$_c$

One possible way to overcome this redundancy may be to consider the capacity qualifier as activity and the performance qualifier as participation.

Another possibility is to develop additional qualifiers for participation that capture "involvement in life situations".

It is expected that with the continued use of ICF and the generation of empirical data, evidence will become available as to which of the above options are preferred by different users of the classification. Empirical research will also lead to a clearer operationalization of the notions of activities and participation. Data on how these notions are used in different settings, in different countries and for different purposes can be generated and will then inform further revisions to the scheme.

Annex 4

Case examples

The examples below describe applications of ICF concepts to various cases. It is hoped that they will assist users to understand the intent and application of the basic classification concepts and constructs. For further details, please refer to WHO training manuals and courses.

Impairment leading to no limitation in capacity and no problem in performance

A child is born with a fingernail missing. This malformation is an impairment of structure, but does not interfere with the function of the child's hand or what the child can do with that hand, so there is no limitation in the child's capacity. Similarly, there may be no performance problem – such as playing with other children without being teased or excluded from play – because of this malformation. The child, therefore, has no capacity limitations or problems in performance.

Impairment leading to no limitation in capacity but to problems in performance

A diabetic child has an impairment of function: the pancreas does not function adequately to produce insulin. Diabetes can be controlled by medication, namely insulin. When the body functions (insulin levels) are under control, there are no limitations in capacity associated with the impairment. However, the child with diabetes is likely to experience a performance problem in socializing with friends or peers when eating is involved, since the child is required to restrict sugar intake. The lack of appropriate food would create a barrier. Therefore, the child would have a lack of involvement in socialisation in the current environment unless steps were taken to ensure that appropriate food was provided, in spite of no limitations in capacity.

Another example is that of an individual with vitiligo on the face but no other physical complaints. This cosmetic problem produces no limitations in capacity. However, the individual may live in a setting where vitiligo is mistaken for leprosy and so considered contagious. In the person's current environment, therefore, this negative attitude is an environmental barrier that leads to significant performance problems in interpersonal interactions.

Impairment leading to limitations in capacity and – depending on circumstance – to problems or no problems in performance

A significant variation in intellectual development is a mental impairment. This may lead to some limitation in a variety of the person's capacities. Environmental factors, however, may affect the extent of the individual's performance in different life domains. For example, a child with this mental impairment might experience little disadvantage in an environment where expectations are not high for the general population and where the child is given an array of simple, repetitive but necessary tasks to accomplish. In this environment the child will perform well in different life situations.

A similar child growing up in an environment of competition and high scholastic expectation might experience more problems in performance in various life situations compared to the first child.

This case example highlights two issues. The first is that the population norm or standard against which an individual's functioning is compared must be appropriate to the actual current environment. The second is that the presence or absence of environmental factors may have either a facilitating or a hindering impact on that functioning.

Former impairment leading to no limitations in capacity but still causing problems in performance

An individual who has recovered from an acute psychotic episode, but who bears the stigma of having been a "mental patient", may experience problems in performance in the domain of employment or interpersonal interactions, because of negative attitudes of people in his or her environment. The person's involvement in employment and social life is, therefore, restricted.

Different impairments and limitations in capacity leading to similar problems in performance

An individual may not be hired for a job because the extent of his or her impairment (quadriplegia) is seen to preclude performing some job requirements (e.g. using a computer with a manual keyboard). The workplace does not have the necessary adaptations to facilitate the person's performance of these job requirements (e.g. voice recognition software that replaces the manual keyboard).

Another individual with less severe quadriplegia may have the capacity to do the necessary job tasks, but may not be hired because the quota for hiring people with disabilities has been filled.

A third individual, who is capable of performing the required job activities, may not be hired because he or she has an activity limitation that is alleviated through use of a wheelchair, although the job site is not accessible to wheelchairs.

Lastly, an individual using a wheelchair may be hired for the job, and has the capacity to do the job tasks and in fact does perform them in the work context. Nonetheless, this individual may still have problems in performing in domains of interpersonal interactions with co-workers, because access to work-related rest areas is not available. This problem of performance in socializing at the place of employment may prevent access to job advancement opportunities.

All four individuals experience performance problems in the domain of employment because of different environmental factors interacting with their health condition or impairment. For the first individual, the environmental barriers include lack of accommodation at the workplace and probably negative attitudes. The second individual is faced with negative attitudes about employment of disabled people. The third person faces lack of accessibility of the built environment and the last person faces negative attitudes about disability generally.

Suspected impairment leading to marked problems in performance without limitations in capacity

An individual has been working with patients who have AIDS. This individual is otherwise healthy but has to undergo periodic testing for HIV. He has no capacity limitations. Despite this, people who know him socially suspect he may have acquired the virus and so avoid him. This leads to significant problems in the person's performance in the domain of social interactions and community, social and civic life. His involvement is restricted because of negative attitudes adopted by the people in his environment.

Impairments currently not classified in ICF leading to problems in performance

An individual has a mother who died of breast cancer. She is 45 years old and was voluntarily screened recently and found to carry the genetic code that puts her at risk for breast cancer. She has no problems in body function or structure, or limitation in capacities, but is denied health insurance by her insurance company because of her increased risk for breast cancer. Her involvement in the domain of looking after her health is restricted because of the policy of the health insurance company.

Additional examples

A 10-year-old boy is referred to a speech therapist with the referral diagnosis "stuttering". During the examination problems are found in discontinuities in speech, inter- and intra-verbal accelerations, problems in timing of speech movements and inadequate speech rhythm (impairments). There are problems at school with reading aloud and with conversation (capacity limitations). During group discussions he does not take any initiative to engage in the discussions although he would like to (performance problem in the domain of conversing with many people). This boy's involvement in conversation is limited when in a group because of societal norms and practices concerning the orderly unfolding of conversations.

A 40-year-old woman with a whiplash injury four months earlier complains about pain in the neck, severe headache, dizziness, reduced muscle power and anxiety (impairments). Her ability to walk, cook, clean, handle a computer and drive a car are limited (limitations in capacity). In consultation with her physician it was mutually agreed to wait till the problems are reduced before she can return to her old full-time fixed-hours job (problems in performance in the domain of employment). If the workplace policies in her current environment allowed for flexible work hours, taking time off when her symptoms were particularly bad, and allowed her to work from home, her involvement in the domain of employment would improve.

Annex 5

ICF and people with disabilities

The ICF revision process has, since its inception, benefited from the input of people with disabilities and organizations of disabled persons. Disabled Peoples' International in particular has contributed its time and energies to the process of revision, and ICF reflects this important input.

WHO recognizes the importance of the full participation of persons with disabilities and their organizations in the revision of a classification of functioning and disability. As a classification, ICF will serve as the basis for both the assessment and measurement of disability in many scientific, clinical, administrative and social policy contexts. As such, it is a matter of concern that ICF not be misused in ways that are detrimental to the interests of persons with disabilities (see Ethical Guidelines in Annex 6).

In particular, WHO recognizes that the very terms used in the classification can, despite the best efforts of all, be stigmatizing and labelling. In response to this concern, the decision was made early in the process to drop the term "handicap" entirely – owing to its pejorative connotations in English – and not to use the term "disability" as the name of a component, but to keep it as the overall, umbrella term.

There remains, however, the difficult question of how best to refer to individuals who experience some degree of functional limitation or restriction. ICF uses the term "disability" to denote a multidimensional phenomenon resulting from the interaction between people and their physical and social environment. For a variety of reasons, when referring to individuals, some prefer to use the term "people with disabilities" while others prefer "disabled people". In the light of this divergence, there is no universal practice for WHO to adopt, and it is not appropriate for ICF rigidly to adopt one rather than another approach. Instead, WHO confirms the important principle that people have the right to be called what they choose.

It is important to stress, moreover, that ICF is not a classification of people at all. It is a classification of people's health characteristics within the context of their individual life situations and environmental impacts. It is the interaction of the health characteristics and the contextual factors that produces disability. This being so, individuals must not be reduced to, or characterized solely in terms of, their impairments, activity limitations, or participation restrictions. For example, instead of referring to a "mentally handicapped person", the classification uses the phrase "person with a problem in learning". ICF ensures this by avoiding any reference to a person by means of a health condition or disability term, and by using neutral, if not positive, and concrete language throughout.

To further address the legitimate concern of systematic labelling of people, the categories in ICF are expressed in a neutral way to avoid depreciation, stigmatization and inappropriate connotations. This approach, however, brings with it the problem of what might be called the "sanitation of terms". The negative attributes of one's health condition and how other people react to it are independent of the terms used to define the condition. Whatever disability is called, it exists irrespective of labels. The problem is not only an issue of language but also, and mainly, an issue of the attitudes of other individuals and society towards disability. What is needed is correct content and usage of terms and classification.

WHO is committed to continuing efforts to ensure that persons with disabilities are empowered by classification and assessment, and not disentitled or discriminated against.

It is hoped that disabled people themselves will contribute to the use and development of ICF in all sectors. As researchers, managers and policy-makers, disabled people will help to develop protocols and tools that are grounded in the ICF classifications. ICF also serves as a potentially powerful tool for evidence-based advocacy. It provides reliable and comparable data to make the case for change. The political notion that disability is as much the result of environmental barriers as it is of health conditions or impairments must be transformed, first into a research agenda and then into valid and reliable evidence. This evidence can bring genuine social change for persons with disabilities around the world.

Disability advocacy can also be enhanced by using ICF. As the primary goal of advocacy is to identify interventions that can improve levels of participation of people with disabilities, ICF can assist in identifying where the principal "problem" of disability lies, whether it is in the environment by way of a barrier or the absence of a facilitator, the limited capacity of the individual himself or herself, or some combination of factors. By means of this clarification, interventions can be appropriately targeted and their effects on levels of participation monitored and measured. In this way, concrete and evidence-driven objectives can be achieved and the overall goals of disability advocacy furthered.

Annex 6

Ethical guidelines for the use of ICF

Every scientific tool can be misused and abused. It would be naive to believe that a classification system such as ICF will never be used in ways that are harmful to people. As explained in Appendix 5, the process of the revision of ICIDH has included persons with disabilities and their advocacy organizations from the beginning. Their input has lead to substantive changes in the terminology, content and structure of ICF. This annex sets out some basic guidelines for the ethical use of ICF. It is obvious that no set of guidelines can anticipate all forms of misuse of a classification or other scientific tool, or for that matter, that guidelines alone can prevent misuse. This document is no exception. It is hoped that attention to the provisions that follow will reduce the risk that ICF will be used in ways that are disrespectful and harmful to people with disabilities.

Respect and confidentiality

(1) ICF should always be used so as to respect the inherent value and autonomy of individual persons.

(2) ICF should never be used to label people or otherwise identify them solely in terms of one or more disability categories.

(3) In clinical settings, ICF should always be used with the full knowledge, cooperation, and consent of the persons whose levels of functioning are being classified. If limitations of an individual's cognitive capacity preclude this involvement, the individual's advocate should be an active participant.

(4) The information coded using ICF should be viewed as personal information and subject to recognized rules of confidentiality appropriate for the manner in which the data will be used.

Clinical use of ICF

(5) Wherever possible, the clinician should explain to the individual or the individual's advocate the purpose of the use of ICF and invite questions about the appropriateness of using it to classify the person's levels of functioning.

(6) Wherever possible, the person whose level of functioning is being classified (or the person's advocate) should have the opportunity to participate, and in particular to challenge or affirm the appropriateness of the category being used and the assessment assigned.

(7) Because the deficit being classified is a result of both a person's health condition and the physical and social context in which the person lives, ICF should be used holistically.

Social use of ICF information

(8) ICF information should be used, to the greatest extent feasible, with the collaboration of individuals to enhance their choices and their control over their lives.

(9) ICF information should be used towards the development of social policy and political change that seeks to enhance and support the participation of individuals.

(10) ICF, and all information derived from its use, should not be employed to deny established rights or otherwise restrict legitimate entitlements to benefits for individuals or groups.

(11) Individuals classed together under ICF may still differ in many ways. Laws and regulations that refer to ICF classifications should not assume more homogeneity than intended and should ensure that those whose levels of functioning are being classified are considered as individuals.

Annex 7

Summary of the revision process

The development of ICIDH

In 1972, WHO developed a preliminary scheme concerning the consequences of disease. Within a few months a more comprehensive approach was suggested. These suggestions were made on two important principles: distinctions were to be made between impairments and their importance, i.e. their functional and social consequences, and these various aspects or axes of the data were to be classified separately in different fields of digits. In essence, this approach consisted of a number of distinct, albeit parallel, classifications. This contrasted with the traditions of ICD, wherein multiple axes (etiology, anatomy, pathology, etc.) are integrated in a hierarchical system occupying only a single field of digits. The possibility of assimilating these proposals into a scheme compatible with the principles underlying the structure of ICD was explored. At the same time, preliminary attempts were made to systematize the terminology applied to disease consequences. These suggestions were circulated informally in 1973, and help was solicited particularly from groups with a special concern in rehabilitation.

Separate classifications for impairments and handicaps were circulated in 1974 and discussions continued. Comments were collated and definitive proposals were developed. These were submitted for consideration by the International Conference for the Ninth Revision of the International Classification of Diseases in October 1975. Having considered the classifications, the Conference recommended its publication for trial purposes. In May 1976, the Twenty-ninth World Health Assembly took note of this recommendation and adopted resolution WHA29.35, in which it approved the publication, for trial purposes, of the supplementary classification of impairments and handicaps as a supplement to, but not as an integral part of, the International Classification of Diseases. Consequently, the first edition of ICIDH was published in 1980. In 1993, it was reprinted with an additional foreword.

Initial steps in the revision of ICIDH

In 1993, it was decided to begin a process of revision of ICIDH. The desiderata for the revised version, know provisionally as ICIDH-2, were as follows:

- it should serve the multiple purposes required by different countries, sectors and health care disciplines;

- it should be simple enough to be seen by practitioners as a meaningful description of consequences of health conditions;

- it should be useful for practice - i.e. identifying health care needs and tailoring intervention programmes (e.g. prevention, rehabilitation, social actions);

- it should give a coherent view of the processes involved in the consequences of health conditions such that the disablement process, and not just the dimensions of diseases/disorders, could be objectively assessed, recorded and responded to;

- it should be sensitive to cultural variations (be translatable, and be applicable in different cultures and health care systems);

- it should be usable in a complementary way with the WHO family of classifications.

Originally, the French Collaborating Centre was given the task of making a proposal on the Impairments section and on language, speech and sensory aspects. The Dutch Collaborating Centre was to suggest a revision of the Disability and locomotor aspects of the Classification and prepare a review of the literature, while the North American Collaborating Centre was to put forward proposals for the Handicap section. In addition, two task forces were to present proposals on mental health aspects and children's issues respectively. Progress was made at a ICIDH-2 revision meeting held in Geneva in 1996, an Alpha draft was collated incorporating the different proposals, and initial pilot testing was conducted. It was decided at the 1996 meeting that each collaborating centre and task force would now be concerned with the draft as a whole and no longer with their former individual areas for revision. From May 1996 to February 1997, the Alpha draft was circulated among collaborating centres and task forces, and comments and suggestions were collated at WHO headquarters. A list of basic questions, setting out the main issues related to the revision, was also circulated in order to facilitate the collection of comments.

The following topics were considered during the process of revision:

- The three-level classification, i.e. Impairments, Disabilities and Handicaps, had been useful and should remain. The inclusion of contextual/ environmental factors should be considered, although most proposals remained at the stage of theoretical development and empirical testing.

- Interrelations between I/D/H and an adequate relationship between them had been an issue for discussion. Many criticisms had pointed to the causal model underlying the 1980 version of ICIDH, the lack of change over time, and the unidirectional flow from impairment to disability to handicap. The revision process had suggested alternative graphic representations.

- ICIDH-1980 was difficult to use. Simplification for use was deemed necessary: the revision should tend towards simplification rather than towards the addition of detail.

- Contextual factors (external – environmental factors / internal – personal factors): these factors, which were major components of the handicap process (as conceptualized in the 1980 version of ICIDH), should be developed as additional schemes within the ICIDH. However, since social and physical factors in the environment and their relationship to Impairments, Disabilities and Handicaps were strongly culture-bound, they should not be a separate dimension within ICIDH. Nevertheless, it was considered that classifications of environmental factors might prove useful in the analysis of national situations and in the development of solutions at the national level.

- Impairments should reflect advances in knowledge of basic biological mechanisms.

- Cultural applicability and universality should be a major aim.

- Development of training and presentation materials was also a major aim of the revision process.

ICIDH-2 Beta-1 and Beta-2 drafts

In March 1997, a Beta-1 draft was produced which integrated the suggestions collected over the previous years. This draft was presented to the ICIDH revision meeting in April 1997. After incorporation of the meeting's decisions the ICIDH-2 Beta-1 draft was issued for field trials in June 1997. Based on all the data and other feedback collected as part of the Beta-1 field trials, a Beta-2 draft was written between January and April 1999. The resulting draft was presented and discussed at the annual meeting on ICIDH-2 in London in April 1999. After incorporation of the meeting's decisions, the Beta-2 draft was printed and issued for field trials in July 1999.

Field trials

The field trials of the Beta-1 draft were conducted from June 1997 to December 1998, and the Beta-2 field trials from July 1999 to September 2000.

The field tests elicited the widest possible participation from WHO Member States and across different disciplines, including sectors such as health insurance, social security, labour, education, and other groups engaged in classifying health conditions (using the International Classification of Diseases, the Nurses' Classification, and the International Standard Classification of Education - ISCED). The aim was to reach a consensus, through clear definitions that were operational. The field trials constituted a continuous process of development, consultation, feedback, updating and testing.

The following studies were conducted as a part of the Beta-1 and Beta-2 field trials:

- translation and linguistic evaluation;
- item evaluation;
- responses to basic question by consensus conferences and individuals;
- feedback from organizations and individuals;
- options testing;
- feasibility and reliability in case evaluations (live or case summaries);
- others (e.g. focus group studies).

The testing focused on cross-cultural and multisectoral issues. More than 50 countries and 1800 experts were involved in the field tests, which have been reported separately.

ICIDH-2 Prefinal version

On the basis of Beta-2 field trial data and in consultation with collaborating centres and the WHO Committee of Experts on Measurement and Classification, the Prefinal version of ICIDH-2 was drafted in October 2000. This draft was presented to a revision meeting in November 2000. Following incorporation of the meeting's recommendations the ICIDH-2 Prefinal version (December 2000) was submitted to the WHO Executive Board in January 2001. The final draft of ICIDH-2 was then presented to the Fifty-fourth World Health Assembly in May 2001.

Endorsement of the final version

After discussion of the final draft, with the title International Classification of Functioning, Disability and Health, the Health Assembly endorsed the new classification in resolution WHA54.21 of 22 May 2001. The resolution reads as follows:

The Fifty-fourth World Health Assembly,

1. ENDORSES the second edition of the International Classification of Impairments, Disabilities and Handicaps (ICIDH), with the title International Classification of Functioning, Disability and Health, henceforth referred to in short as ICF;

2. URGES Member States to use the ICF in their research, surveillance and reporting as appropriate, taking into account specific situations in Member States and, in particular, in view of possible future revisions;

3. REQUESTS the Director-General to provide support to Member States, at their request, in making use of ICF.

Annex 8

Future directions for ICF

Use of ICF will largely depend on its practical utility: the extent to which it can serve as a measure of health service performance through indicators based on consumer outcomes, and the degree to which it is applicable across cultures so that international comparisons can be made to identify needs and resources for planning and research. ICF is not directly a political tool. Its use may, however, contribute positive input to policy determination by providing information to help establish health policy, promote equal opportunities for all people, and support the fight against discrimination based on disability.

Versions of ICF

In view of the differing needs of different types of users, ICF will be presented in multiple formats and versions.

Main classification

The two parts and their components in ICF are presented in two versions in order to meet the needs of different users for varying levels of detail:

The first version is a *full (detailed) version* which provides all levels of classification and allows for 9999 categories per component. However, a much smaller number of them have been used. The full version categories can be aggregated into the short version when summary information is required.

The second version is a *short (concise) version* which gives two levels of categories for each component and domain. Definitions of these terms, inclusions and exclusions are also given.

Specific adaptations

(a) Clinical use versions: these versions will depend on the use of ICF in different clinical application fields (e.g. occupational therapy). They will be based on the main volume for coding and terminology; however, they will provide further detailed information such as guidelines for assessment and clinical descriptions. They can also be rearranged for specific disciplines (e.g. rehabilitation, mental health).

(b) Research versions: in a similar way to the clinical versions, these versions will respond to specific research needs and will provide precise and operational definitions to assess conditions.

Future work

Given the multitude of uses and needs for ICF, it is important to note that WHO and its collaborating centres are conducting additional work to meet those needs.

ICF is owned by all its users. It is the only such tool accepted on an international basis. It aims to obtain better information on disability phenomena and functioning and build a broad international consensus. To achieve recognition of ICF by various national and international communities, WHO has made every effort to ensure that it is user-friendly and compatible with standardization processes such as those laid down by the International Organization for Standardization (ISO).

The possible future directions for development and application of ICF can be summarized as follows:

- promoting use of ICF at country-level for the development of national databases;

- establishing an international data set and a framework to permit international comparisons;

- identification of algorithms for eligibility for social benefits and pensions;

- study of disability and functioning of family members (e.g. a study of third-party disability due to the health condition of significant others);

- development of a Personal Factors component;

- development of precise operational definitions of categories for research purposes;

- development of assessment instruments for identification and measurement;[29]

- providing practical applications by means of computerization and case-recording forms;

- establishing links with quality-of-life concepts and the measurement of subjective well-being;[30]

- research into treatment or intervention matching;

- promoting use in scientific studies for comparison between different health conditions;

- development of training materials on the use of ICF;

- creation of ICF training and reference centres worldwide.

- further research on environmental factors to provide the necessary detail for use in describing both the standardized and current environment.

---

[29] Assessment instruments linked to ICF are being developed by WHO with a view to applicability in different cultures. They are being tested for reliability and validity.
Assessment instruments will take three forms: a brief version for screening/case-finding purposes; a version for daily use by care-givers; and a long version for detailed research purposes. They will be available from WHO.

[30] Links with quality of life: it is important that there is conceptual compatibility between "quality of life" and disability constructs. Quality of life, however, deals with what people "feel" about their health condition or its consequences; hence it is a construct of "subjective well-being". On the other hand, disease/disability constructs refer to objective and exteriorized signs of the individual.

Annex 9

Suggested ICF data requirements for ideal and minimal health information systems or surveys

Body Functions and Structures	Chapter and code		Classification block or category
Vision	2	b210–b220	Seeing and related functions
Hearing	2	b230–b240	Hearing and vestibular functions
Speech	3	b310–b340	Voice and speech functions
Digestion	5	b510–b535	Functions of the digestive system
Bodily excretion	6	b610–b630	Urinary functions
Fertility	6	b640–b670	Genital and reproductive functions
Sexual activity	6	b640	Genital and reproductive health
Skin and disfigurement	8	b810–b830	Skin and related structures
Breathing	4	b440–b460	Functions of the respiratory system
Pain*	2	b280	Pain
Affect*	1	b152–b180	Specific mental functions
Sleep	1	b134	Global mental functions
Energy/vitality	1	b130	Global mental functions
Cognition*	1	b140, b144, b164	Attention, memory and higher-level cognitive functions
Activities and Participation			
Communication	3	d310–d345	Communication receiving – producing
Mobility*	4	d450–d465	Walking and moving
Dexterity	4	d430–d445	Carrying, moving and handling objects
Self-care*	5	d510–d570	Self-care
Usual activities*	6 and 8		Domestic life; Major life areas
Interpersonal relations	7	d730–d770	Particular interpersonal relationships
Social functioning	9	d910–d930	Community social and civic life

---

*Candidate items for a minimal list.

Appendix 10

Acknowledgements

The development of ICF would not have been possible without the extensive support of many people from different parts of the world who have devoted a great amount of time and energy and organized resources within an international network. While it may not be possible to acknowledge them all here, leading centres, organizations and individuals are listed below.

WHO Collaborating Centres for ICF

Australia	Australian Institute of Health and Welfare, GPO Box 570, Canberra ACT 2601, Australia. Contact: Ros Madden.
Canada	Canadian Institute for Health Information, 377 Dalhousie Street, Suite 200, Ottawa, Ontario KIN9N8, Canada. Contact: Helen Whittome.
France	Centre Technique National d`Etudes et de Recherches sur les Handicaps et les Inadaptations (CTNERHI), 236 bis, rue de Tolbiac, 75013 Paris, France. Contact: Marc Maudinet.
Japan	Japan College of Social Work, 3-1-30 Takeoka, Kiyose-city, Tokyo 204-8555, Japan. Contact: Hisao Sato.
Netherlands	National Institute of Public Health and the Environment, Department of Public Health Forecasting, Antonie van Leeuwenhoeklaan 9, P.O. Box 1, 3720 BA Bilthoven, The Netherlands. Contacts: Willem M. Hirs, Marijke W. de Kleijn-de Vrankrijker.
Nordic countries	Department of Public Health and Caring Sciences, Uppsala Science Park, SE 75185 Uppsala, Sweden. Contact: Björn Smedby.
United Kingdom of Great Britain and Northern Ireland	National Health System Information Authority, Coding and Classification, Woodgate, Loughborough, Leics LE11 2TG, United Kingdom. Contacts: Ann Harding, Jane Millar.
United States of America	National Center for Health Statistics, Room 1100, 6525 Belcrest Road, Hyattsville MD 20782, USA. Contact: Paul J. Placek.

Task forces

International Task Force on Mental Health and Addictive, Behavioural, Cognitive, and Developmental Aspects of ICIDH, Chair: Cille Kennedy, Office of Disability, Aging and Long-Term Care Policy, Office of the Assistant Secretary for Planning and Evaluation,

Department of Health and Human Services, 200 Independence Avenue, SW, Room 424E, Washington, DC 20201, USA. Co-Chair: Karen Ritchie.

Children and Youth Task Force, Chair: Rune J. Simeonsson, Professor of Education, Frank Porter Graham Child Development Center, CB # 8185, University of North Carolina, Chapel Hill, NC 27599-8185, USA. Co-Chair: Matilde Leonardi.

Environmental Factors Task Force, Chair: Rachel Hurst, 11 Belgrave Road, London SW1V 1RB, England. Co-Chair: Janice Miller.

Networks

La Red de Habla Hispana en Discapacidades (The Spanish Network). Coordinator: José Luis Vázquez-Barquero, Unidad de Investigacion en Psiquiatria Clinical y Social Hospital Universitario "Marques de Valdecilla", Avda. Valdecilla s/n, Santander 39008, Spain.

Council of Europe Committee of Experts for the Application of ICIDH, Council of Europe, F-67075, Strasbourg, France. Contact: Lauri Sivonen.

Nongovernmental organizations

American Psychological Association, 750 First Street, N.E., Washington, DC 20002-4242, USA. Contacts: Geoffrey M. Reed, Jayne B. Lux.

Disabled Peoples International, 11 Belgrave Road, London SW1V 1RB, England. Contact: Rachel Hurst.

European Disability Forum, Square Ambiorix, 32 Bte 2/A, B-1000, Bruxelles, Belgium. Contact: Frank Mulcahy.

European Regional Council for the World Federation of Mental Health (ERCWFM), Blvd Clovis N.7, 1000 Brussels, Belgium. Contact: John Henderson.

Inclusion International, 13D Chemin de Levant, F-01210 Ferney-Voltaire, France. Contact: Nancy Breitenbach

Rehabilitation International, 25 E. 21st Street, New York, NY 10010, USA. Contact: Judith Hollenweger, Chairman, RI Education Commission, Institute of Special Education, University of Zurich, Hirschengraben 48, 8001 Zurich, Switzerland.

Consultants

A number of WHO consultants provided invaluable assistance in the revision process. They are listed below.

Elizabeth Badley

Jerome E. Bickenbach

Nick Glozier

Judith Hollenweger

Cille Kennedy

Jane Millar

Janice Miller

Jürgen Rehm

Robin Room

Angela Roberts

Michael F. Schuntermann

Robert Trotter II

David Thompson (editorial consultant)

Translation of ICF in WHO official languages

ICF has been revised in multiple languages taking English as a working language only. Translation and linguistic analysis have been integral part of the revision process. The following WHO collaborators have lead the translation, linguistic analyses, editorial review the WHO official languages. Other translations can be found on the WHO web site: http://www.who.int/classifications/icf.

Arabic

Translation and linguistic analysis:
> Adel Chaker, Ridha Limem, Najeh Daly, Hayet Baachaoui, Amor Haji, Mohamed Daly, Jamil Taktak, Saïda Douki

Editorial review carried out by WHO/EMRO:
> Kassem Sara, M. Haytham Al Khayat, Abdel Aziz Saleh

Chinese

Translation and linguistic analysis:
> Qiu Zhuoying (co-ordinator), Hong Dong, Zhao Shuying, Li Jing, Zhang Aimin, Wu Xianguang, Zhou Xiaonan

Editorial review carried out by WHO Collaborating Centre in China and WHO/WPRO:
> Dong Jingwu, Zhou Xiaonan and Y.C. Chong

French

Translation and linguistic analysis carried out by WHO Geneva:
> Pierre Lewalle

Editorial review carried out by WHO Collaborating Centres in France and Canada:
Catherine Barral and Janice Miller

Russian

Translation and linguistic analysis:
G. Shostka (Co-ordinator), Vladimir Y. Ryasnyansky, Alexander V. Kvashin, Sergey A. Matveev, Aleksey A. Galianov

Editorial review carried out by WHO Collaborating Centre in Russia:
Vladimir K. Ovcharov

Spanish

Translation, linguistic analysis, editorial review by the Collaborating Centre in Spain in collaboration with La Red de Habla Hispana en Discapacidades (The Spanish Network) and WHO/PAHO:
J. L. Vázquez-Barquero (Co-ordinator), Ana Díez Ruiz, Luis Gaite Pindado, Ana Gómez Silió, Sara Herrera Castanedo, Marta Uriarte Ituiño, Elena Vázquez Bourgon Armando Vásquez, María del Consuelo Crespo, Ana María Fossatti Pons, Benjamín Vicente, Pedro Rioseco, Sergio Aguilar Gaxiola, Carmen Lara Muñoz, María Elena Medina Mora, María Esther Araujo Bazán, Carlos Castillo-Salgado, Roberto Becker, Margaret Hazlewood

Individual participants in the revision process

Argentina
Liliana Lissi
Martha Adela Mazas
Miguela Pico
Ignacio Saenz

Armenia
Armen Sargsyan

Australia
Gavin Andrews
Robyne Burridge
Ching Choi
Prem K. Chopra
Jeremy Couper
Elisabeth Davis
Maree Dyson
Rhonda Galbally
Louise Golley
Tim Griffin
Simon Haskell
Angela Hewson
Tracie Hogan
Richard Madden
Ros Madden
Helen McAuley
Trevor Parmenter
Mark Pattison
Tony M. Pinzone
Kate Senior
Catherine Sykes
John Taplin
John Walsh

Austria
Gerhard S. Barolin
Klemens Fheodoroff
Christiane Meyer-
Bornsen

Belgium
Françoise Jan
Catherine Mollman
J. Stevens
A. Tricot

Brazil
Cassia Maria Buchalla

E. d'Arrigo Busnello
Ricardo Halpern
Fabio Gomes
Ruy Laurenti

Canada
Hugh Anton
J. Arboleda-Florez
Denise Avard
Elizabeth Badley
Caroline Bergeron

Hélène Bergeron
Jerome E. Bickenbach
Andra Blanchet
Maurice Blouin
Mario Bolduc
(deceased)
Lucie Brosseau
T.S. Callanan
Lindsay Campbell
Anne Carswell
Jacques Cats
L.S. Cherry
René Cloutier
Albert Cook
Jacques Côté
Marcel Côté
Cheryl Cott
Aileen Davis
Henry Enns
Gail Finkel
Christine Fitzgerald
Patrick Fougeyrollas
Adele Furrie
Linda Garcia
Yhetta Gold
Betty Havens
Anne Hébert
Peter Henderson
Lynn Jongbloed
Faith Kaplan
Ronald Kaplan
Lee Kirby
Catherine Lachance
Jocelyne Lacroix
Renée Langlois
Mary Law

Lucie Lemieux-
Brassard
Annette Majnemer
Rose Martini
Raoul Martin-Blouin
Mary Ann McColl
Joan McComas
Barbara McElgunn
Janice Miller
Louise Ogilvie
Luc Noreau
Diane Richler
Laurie Ringaert
Kathia Roy
Patricia Sisco
Denise Smith
Ginette St Michel
Debra Stewart
Luz Elvira Vallejo
Echeverri
Michael Wolfson
Sharon Wood-
Dauphinee
Nancy Young
Peter Wass
Colleen Watters

Chile
Ricardo Araya
Alejandra Faulbaum
Luis Flores
Roxane Moncayo de
Bremont
Pedro Rioseco
Benjamin Vicente

China
Zhang Aimin
Mary Chu Manlai
Hong Dong
Leung Kwokfai
Karen Ngai Ling
Wu Xuanguong
Qiu Zhuoying
Zhao Shuying
Li Jing
Tang Xiaoquan
Li Jianjun

Ding Buotan
Zhuo Dahong
Nan Dengkun
Zhou Xiaonan

Colombia
Martha Aristabal
Gomez

Côte d'Ivoire
B. Claver

Croatia
Ana Bobinac-
Georgievski

Cuba
Pedro Valdés Sosa
Jesús Saiz Sánchez
Frank Morales
Aguilera

Denmark
Terkel Andersen
Aksel Bertelsen
Tora Haraldsen Dahl
Marianne Engberg
Annette Flensborg
Ane Fink
Per Fink
Lise From
Jette Haugbølle
Stig Langvad
Lars von der Lieth
Kurt Møller
Claus Vinther Nielsen
Freddy Nielsen
Kamilla Rothe Nissen
Gunnar Schiøler
Anne Sloth
Susan Tetler
Selena Forchhammer
Thønnings
Eva Wæhrens
Brita Øhlenschlæger

Ecuador
María del Consuelo
Crespo
Walter Torres

Izquierdo

Egypt
Mohammed El-Banna

El Salvador
Jorge Alberto Alcarón
Patricia Tovar de
Canizalez

Ethiopia
Rene Rakotobe

Finland
Erkki Yrjankeikki
Markku Leskinen
Leena Matikka
Matti Ojala
Heidi Paatero
Seija Talo
Martti Virtanen

France
Charles Aussilloux
Bernard Azema
Jacques Baert
Serge Bakchine
Catherine Barral
Maratine Barres
Jean-Yves Barreyre
Jean-Paul Boissin
François Chapireau
Pascal Charpentier
Alain Colvez
Christian Corbé
Dr. Cyran
Michel Delcey
Annick Deveau
Serge Ebersold
Camille Felder
Claude Finkelstein
Anne-Marie Gallot
Pascale Gilbert
Jacques Houver
Marcel Jaeger
Jacques Jonquères
Jean-Claude Lafon
Maryvonne Lyazid
Joëlle Loste-Berdot
Maryse Marrière

Lucie Matteodo
Marc Maudinet
Jean-Michel Mazeaux
Pierre Minaire *(deceased)*
Lucien Moatti
Bertrand Morineaux
Pierre Mormiche
Jean-Michel Orgogozo
Claudine Parayre
Gérard Pavillon
André Philip
Nicole Quemada
Jean-François Ravaud
Karen Ritchie
Jean-Marie Robine
Isabelle Romieu
Christian Rossignol
Pascale Roussel
Jacques Roustit
Jésus Sanchez
Marie-José Schmitt
Jean-Luc Simon
Lauri Sivonen
Henri-Jacques Stiker
Annie Triomphe
Catherine Vaslin
Paul Veit
Dominique Velche
Jean-Pierre Vignat
Vivian Waltz

Germany
Helmi Böse-Younes
Horst Dilling
Thomas Ewert
Kurt Maurer
Jürgen Rehm
H.M. Schian
Michael F.
Schuntermann
Ute Siebel
Gerold Stucki

Greece
Venos Mavreas

Hungary
Lajos Kullmann

India
Javed Abidi
Samir Guha-Roy
K.S. Jacob
Sunanda Koli
S. Murthy
D.M. Naidu
Hemraj Pal
K. Sekar
K.S. Shaji
Shobha Srinath
T.N. Srinivasan
R. Thara

Indonesia
Augustina Hendriarti

Iran (Islamic Republic of)
Mohamed M.R.
Mourad

Israel
Joseph Yahav

Italy
Emilio Alari
Alberto Albanese
Renzo Andrich
A.Andrigo
Andrea Arrigo
Marco Barbolini
Maurizio Bejor
Giulio Borgnolo
Gabriella Borri
Carlo Caltagirone
Felicia Carletto
Carla Colombo
Francesca Cretti
Maria Cufersin
Marta Dao
Mario D'Amico
Simona Della Bianca
Paolo Di Benedetto
Angela Di Lorenzo
Nadia Di Monte
Vittoria Dieni
Antonio Federico
Francesco Fera
Carlo Francescutti
Francesca Fratello

Franco Galletti
Federica Galli
Rosalia Gasparotto
Maria Teresa Gattesco
Alessandro
Giacomazzi
Tullio Giorgini
Elena Giraudo
Lucia Granzini
Elena Grosso
V. Groppo
Vincenzo Guidetti
Paolo Guzzon
Leo Giulio Iona
Vladimir Kosic
Matilde Leonardi
Fulvia Loik
Mariangela Macan
Alessandra Manassero
Domenico Manco
Santina Mancuso
Roberto Marcovich
Andrea Martinuzzi
Anna Rosa Melodia
Rosetta Mussari
Cristiana Muzzi
Ugo Nocentini
Emanuela Nogherotto
Roberta Oretti
Lorenzo Panella
Maria Procopio
Leandro Provinciali
Alda Pellegri
Barbara Reggiori
Marina Sala
Giorgio Sandrini
Antonio Schindler
Elena Sinforiani
Stefano Schierano
Roberto Sicurelli
Francesco Talarico
Gariella Tavoschi
Cristiana Tiddia
Walter Tomazzoli
Corrado Tosetto
Sergio Ujcich
Maria Rosa Valsecchi
Irene Vernero

Jamaica
Monica Bartley

Japan
Tsunehiko Akamatsu
Masataka Arima
Hidenobu Fujisono
Katsunori Fujita
Shinichiro Furuno
Toshiko Futaki
Hajime Hagiwara
Yuichiro Haruna
Hideaki Hyoudou
Takashi Iseda
Atsuko Ito
Shinya Iwasaki
Shizuko Kawabata
Yasu Kiryu
Akira Kodama
Ryousuke Matsui
Ryo Matsutomo
Yasushi Mochizuki
Kazuyo Nakai
Kenji Nakamura
Yoshukuni Nakane
Yukiko Nakanishi
Toshiko Niki
Hidetoshi Nishijima
Shiniti Niwa
Kensaku Ohashi
Mari Oho
Yayoi Okawa
Shuhei Ota
Fumiko Rinko
Junko Sakano
Yoshihiko Sasagawa
Hisao Sato
Yoshiyuki Suzuki
Junko Taguchi
Eiichi Takada
Yuji Takagi
Masako Tateishi
Hikaru Tauchi
Miyako Tazaki
Mutsuo Torai
Satoshi Ueda
Kousuke Yamazaki
Yoshio Yazaki

Jordan
Abdulla S.T. El-
Naggar
Ziad Subeih

Kuwait
Adnan Al Eidan
Abdul Aziz Khalaf
Karam

Latvia
Valda Biedrina
Aldis Dudins
Lolita Cibule
Janis Misins
Jautrite Karashkevica
Mara Ozola
Aivars Vetra

Lebanon
Elie Karam

Lithuania
Albinas Bagdonas

Luxembourg
Charles Pull
M. De Smedt
Pascale Straus

Malaysia
Sandiyao Sebastian

Madagascar
Caromène
Ratomahenina
Raymond

Malta
Joe M. Pace

Mexico
Juan Alberto
Alcantara
Jorge Caraveo
Anduaga
María Eugenia
Antunez
Fernando R. Jiménez
Albarran

Gloria Martinez
Carrera
María-Elena Medina
Mora
Carmen E. Lara
Muñoz

Morocco
Aziza Bennani

Netherlands
T. van Achterberg
Jaap van den Berg
A. Bloemhof
Y.M. van der Brug
R.D. de Boer
J.T.P. Bonte
J.W. Brandsma
W.H.E. Buntinx
J.P.M. Diederiks
M J Driesse
Silvia van Duuren-
Kristen
C.M.A. Frederiks
J.C. Gerritse
José Geurts
G. Gladines
K.A. Gorter
R.J. de Haan
J. Halbertsma
E.J. van der Haring
F.G. Hellema
C.H. Hens-Versteeg
Y. F. Heerkens
Y. Heijnen
W.M. Hirs
H. W. Hoek
D. van Hoeken
N. Hoeymans
C. van Hof
G.R.M. van Hoof
M. Hopman-Rock
A. Kap
E.J. Karel
Zoltan E. Kenessey
M.C.O. Kersten
M.W. de Kleijn-de
Vrankrijker
M.M.Y. de Klerk

M. Koenen
J.W. Koten
D.W.Kraijer
T. Kraakman
Guuss Lankhorst
W.A.L. van Leeuwen
P. Looijestein
H. Meinardi
W. van Minnen
A.E. Monteny
I. Oen
Wil Ooijendijk
W.J. den Ouden
R.J.M. Perenboom
A. Persoon
J.J. v.d. Plaats
M. Poolmans
F.J. Prinsze
C.D. van Ravensberg
K. Reynders
K. Riet-van Hoof
G. Roodbol
G.L. Schut
B. Stoelinga
M.M.L. Swart
L. Taal
H. Ten Napel
B. Treffers
J. Verhoef
A. Vermeer
J.J.G.M. Verwer
W. Vink
M. Welle Donker
Dirk Wiersma
J.P. Wilken
P.A. van Woudenberg
P.H.M. Wouters
P. Zanstra

Nicaragua
Elizabeth Aguilar
Angel Bonilla Serrano
Ivette Castillo
Héctor Collado
Hernández
Josefa Conrado
Brenda Espinoza
María Félix Gontol
Mirian Gutiérrez

Rosa Gutiérrez
Carlos Guzmán
Luis Jara
Raúl Jarquin
Norman Lanzas
José R. Leiva
Rafaela Marenco
María Alejandra
Martínez
Marlon Méndez
Mercedes Mendoza
María José Moreno
Alejandra Narváez
Amilkar Obando
Dulce María Olivas
Rosa E. Orellana
Yelba Rosa Orozco
Mirian Ortiz Alvarado
Amanda Pastrana
Marbely Picado
Susana Rappaciolli
Esterlina Reyes
Franklin Rivera
Leda María Rodríguez
Humberto Román
Yemira Sequeira
Ivonne Tijerino
Ena Liz Torrez
Rene Urbina
Luis Velásquez

Nigeria
Sola Akinbiyi
John Morakinyo
A. O. Odejide
Olayinka Omigbodun

Norway
Kjetil Bjorlo
Torbjorg Hostad
Kjersti Vik
Nina Vollestad
Margret Grotle
Soukup
Sigrid Ostensjo

Pakistan
S. Khan
Malik H. Mubbashar
Khalid Saeed

Philippines
L. Ladrigo-Ignacio
Patria Medina

Peru
María Esther Araujo
Bazon
Carlos Bejar Vargas
Carmen Cifuentes
Granados
Roxana Cock Huaman
Lily Pinguz Vergara
Adriana Rebaza Flores
Nelly Roncal Velazco
Fernando Urcia
Fernández
Rosa Zavallos Piedra

Republic of Korea
Ack-Seop Lee

Romania
Radu Vrasti

Russia
Vladimir N. Blondin
Aleksey A. Galianov
I.Y. Gurovich
Mikhail V. Korobov
Alexander V.
Kvashin
Pavel A.
Makkaveysky
Sergey A. Matveev
N. Mazaeva
Vladimir K.
Ovtcharov
S.V. Polubinskaya
Anna G. Ryabokon
Vladimir Y.
Ryasnyansky
Alexander V. Shabrov
Georgy D. Shostka
Sergei Tsirkin
Yuri M. Xomarov
Alexander Y.
Zemtchenkov

Slovenia
Andreeja Fatur-

Videtec

South Africa
David Boonzaier
Gugulethu Gule
Sebenzile Matsebula
Pam McLaren
Siphokazi Gcaza
Phillip Thompson

Spain
Alvaro Bilbao Bilbao
Encarnación Blanco
Egido
Rosa Bravo Rodriguez
María José Cabo
González
Marta Cano Fernández
Laura Cardenal
Villalba
Ana Diez Ruiz
Luis Gaite Pindado
María García José
Ana Gómez Silió
Andres Herran Gómez
Sara Herrera
Castanedo
Ismael Lastra
Martinez
Marta Uriarte Ituiño
Elena Vázquez
Bourgon
Antonio León Aguado
Díaz
Carmen Albeza
Contreras
María Angeles Aldana
Berberana
Federico Alonso
Trujillo
Carmen Alvarez
Arbesú
Jesus Artal Simon
Enrique Baca
Baldomero
Julio Bobes García
Antonio Bueno
Alcántara
Tomás Castillo Arenal

Valentín Corces
Pando
María Teresa Crespo
Abelleira
Roberto Cruz
Hernández
José Armando De
Vierna Amigo
Manuel Desviat
Muñoz
Ana María Díaz
García
María José Eizmendi
Apellaniz
Antonio Fernández
Moral
Manuel A. Franco
Martín
Luis Gaite Pinadado
María Mar García
Amigo
José Giner-Ubago
Gregorio Gómez-
Jarabo
José Manuel Gorospe
Arocena
Juana María
Hernández Rodríguez
Carmen Leal Cercos
Marcelino López
Alvarez
Juan José Lopez-Ibor
Ana María López
Trenco
Francisco Margallo
Polo
Monica Martín Gil
Miguel Martín
Zurimendi
Manuel J. Martínez
Cardeña
Juan Carlos
Miangolarra Page
Rosa M.Montoliu
Valls
Teresa Orihuela
Villameriel
Sandra Ortega Mera
Gracia Parquiña

Fernández
Rafael Peñalver
Castellano
Jesusa Pertejo
María Francisca
Peydro de Moya
Juan Rafael Prieto
Lucena
Miguel Querejeta
González
Miquel Roca Bennasar
Francisco Rodríguez
Pulido
Luis Salvador Carulla
María Vicenta
Sánchez de la Cruz
Francisco Torres
González
María Triquell Manuel
José Luis Vázquez-
Barquero
Miguel A.Verdugo
Alonso
Carlos Villaro Díaz-
Jiménez

Sweden
Lars Berg
Eva Bjorck-Akesson
Mats Granlund
Gunnar Grimby
Arvid Linden
Anna Christina Nilson
(deceased)
Anita Nilsson
Louise Nilunger
Lennart Nordenfelt
Adolf Ratzka
Gunnar Sanner
Olle Sjögren
Björn Smedby
Sonja Calais van
Stokkom
Gabor Tiroler

Switzerland
André
Assimacopoulos
Christoph Heinz

Judith Hollenweger
Hans Peter Rentsch
Thomas Spuhler
Werner Steiner
John Strome
John-Paul Vader
Peter Wehrli
Rudolf Widmer

Thailand
Poonpit Amatuakul
Pattariya Jarutat
C. Panpreecha
K. Roongruangmaairat
Pichai Tangsin

Tunisia
Adel Chaker
Hayet Baachaoui
A. Ben Salem
Najeh Daly
Saïda Douki
Ridha Limam
Mhalla Nejia
Jamil Taktak

Turkey
Ahmet Gögüs
Elif Iyriboz
Kultegin Ogel
Berna Ulug

United Arab Emirates
Sheika Jamila Bint Al-
Qassimi

**United Kingdom of Great
Britain and Northern
Ireland**
Simone Aspis
Allan Colver
Edna Conlan
John E. Cooper
A. John Fox
Nick Glozier
Ann Harding
Rachel Hurst
Rachel Jenkins
Howard Meltzer
Jane Millar

Peter Mittler
Martin Prince
Angela Roberts
G. Stewart
Wendy Thorne
Andrew Walker
Brian Williams

United States of America
Harvey Abrams
Myron J. Adams
Michelle Adler
Sergio A. Aguilor-
Gaxiola
Barbara Altman
Alicia Amate
William Anthony
Susan Spear Basset
Frederica Barrows
Mark Battista
Robert Battjes
Barbara Beck
Karin Behe
Cynthia D. Belar
J.G. Benedict
Stanley Berent
Linas Bieliauskas
Karen Blair
F. Bloch
Felicia Hill Briggs
Edward P. Burke
Larry Burt
Shane S. Bush
Glorisa Canino
Jean Campbell
Scott Campbell Brown
John A. Carpenter
Christine H.
Carrington
Judi Chamberlin
LeeAnne Carrothers
Mary Chamie
Cecelia B. Collier
William Connors
John Corrigan
Dale Cox
M. Doreen Croser
Eugene D'Angelo
Gerben DeJong

Jeffrey E. Evans
Timothy G. Evans
Debbie J. Farmer
Michael Feil
Manning Feinleib
Risa Fox
Carol Frattali
Bill Frey
E. Fuller
Cheryl Gagne
J. Luis Garcia Segura
David W. Gately
Carol George
Olinda Gonzales
Barbara Gottfried
Bridget Grant
Craig Gray
David Gray
Marjorie Greenberg
Arlene Greenspan
Frederick
Guggenheim
Neil Hadder
Harlan Hahn
Robert Haines
Laura Lee Hall
Heather Hancock
Nandini Hawley
Gregory W. Heath
Gerry Hendershot
Sarah Hershfeld
Sarah Hertfelder
Alexis Henry
Howard Hoffman
Audrey Holland
Joseph G. Hollowell Jr
Andrew Imparato
John Jacobson
Judith Jaeger
Alan Jette
J. Rock Johnson
Gisele Kamanou-
Goune
Charles Kaelber
Cille Kennedy
Donald G. Kewman
Michael Kita (*deceased*)
Edward Knight
Pataricia Kricos

Susan Langmore
Mitchell LaPlante
Itzak Levav
Renee Levinson
Robert Liberman
Don Lollar
Peter Love
David Lozovsky
Perianne Lurie
Jayne B. Lux
Reid Lyon
Anis Maitra
Bob MacBride
Kim MacDonald-
Wilson
Peggy Maher
Ronald Manderscheid
Kofi Marfo
Ana Maria
Margueytio
William C. Marrin
John Mather
Maria Christina
Mathiason
John McGinley
Theresa McKenna
Christine McKibbin
Christopher J.
McLaughlin
Laurie McQueen
Douglas Moul
Peter E. Nathan
Russ Newman
Els R. Nieuwenhuijsen
Joan F. van Nostrand
Jean Novak
Patricia Owens
Alcida Perez de
Velasquez
D. Jesse Peters
David B. Peterson
Harold Pincus
Paul Placek
Thomas E. Preston
Maxwell Prince
Jeffrey Pyne
Louis Quatrano
Juan Ramos
Geoffrey M. Reed

Anne Riley
Gilberto Romero
Patricia Roberts-Rose
Mark A. Sandberg
Judy Sangl
Marian Scheinholtz
Karin Schumacher
Katherine D. Seelman
Raymond Seltser
Rune J. Simeonsson
Debra Smith
Gretchen Swanson
Susan Stark
Denise G. Tate
Travis Threats
Cynthia Trask
Robert Trotter II
R. Alexander Vachon
Maureen Valente
Paolo del Vecchio
Lois Verbrugge

Katherine Verdolini
Candace Vickers
Gloriajean Wallace
Robert Walsh
Seth A. Warshausky
Paul Weaver
Patricia Welch
Gale Whiteneck
Tyler Whitney
Brian Williams
Jan Williams
Linda Wornall
J. Scott Yaruss
Ilene Zeitzer
Louise Zingeser

Uruguay
Paulo Alterway
Marta Barera
Margot Barrios
Daniela Bilbao

Gladys Curbelo
Ana M. Frappola
Ana M. Fosatti Pons
Angélica Etcheñique
Rosa Gervasio
Mariela Irigoin
Fernando Lavie
Silvia Núñez
Rossana Pipplol
Silvana Toledo

Vietnam
Nguyen Duc Truyen

Zimbabwe
Jennifer Jelsma
Dorcas Madzivire
Gillian Marks
Jennifer Muderedzi
Useh Ushotanefe

Organizations of the United Nations system

International Labour Organization (ILO)
Susan Parker

United Nations Children's Fund (UNICEF)
Habibi Gulbadan

United Nations Statistical Division
Margarat Mbogoni
Joann Vanek

United Nations Statistical Institute for Asia and the Pacific
Lau Kak En

United Nations Economic and Social Commission for Asia and
Pacific
Bijoy Chaudhari

World Health Organization

Regional Offices

Africa: C. Mandlhate

Americas (Pan American Health Organisation): Carlos Castillo-Salgado,
Roberto Becker, Margaret Hazlewood, Armando Vázquez

Eastern Mediterranean: A. Mohit, Abdel Aziz Saleh, Kassem Sara, M. Haytham Al Khayat

Europe: B. Serdar Savas, Anatoli Nossikov

South-East Asia: Than Sein, Myint Htwe

Western Pacific: R. Nesbit, Y.C. Chong

Headquarters

Various departments at WHO headquarters were involved in the revision process. Individual staff members who contributed to the revision process are listed below with their departments are listed below.

M. Argandoña, formerly of Department of Substance Abuse

Z. Bankowski, Council for International Organizations of Medical Sciences

J.A. Costa e Silva, formerly Division of Mental Health and Prevention of Substance Abuse

S. Clark, Department of Health Information, Management and Dissemination

C. Djeddah, Department of Injuries and Violence Prevention

A. Goerdt, formerly of Department of Health Promotion

M. Goracci, formerly of Department of Injury Prevention and Rehabilitation

M. A. Jansen, formerly of Department of Mental Health and Substance Dependence

A. L'Hours, Global Programme on Evidence for Health Policy

A. Lopez, Global Programme on Evidence for Health Policy

J. Matsumoto, Department of External Cooperation and Partnerships

C. Mathers, Global Programme on Evidence for Health Policy

C. Murray, Global Programme on Evidence for Health Policy

H. Nabulsi, formerly of IMPACT

E. Pupulin, Department of Management of Noncommunicable Diseases

C. Romer, Department of Injuries and Violence Prevention

R. Sadana, Global Programme on Evidence for Health Policy

B. Saraceno, Department of Mental Health and Substance Dependence

A. Smith, Department of Management of Noncommunicable Diseases

J. Salomon, Global Programme on Evidence for Health Policy

M. Subramanian, formerly of World Health Reporting

M. Thuriaux, formerly of Division of Emerging and other Communicable Diseases

B. Thylefors, formerly of Department of Disability/Injury Prevention and Rehabilitation

M. Weber, Department of Child and Adolescent Health and Development

Sibel Volkan and Grazia Motturi provided administrative and secretarial support.

Can Çelik, Pierre Lewalle, Matilde Leonardi, Senda Bennaissa and Luis Prieto carried out specific aspects of the revision work.

Somnath Chatterji, Shekhar Saxena, Nenad Kostanjsek and Margie Schneider carried out the revision based on all the inputs received.

T. Bedirhan Üstün managed and coordinated the revision process and the overall ICF project.

ICF-CY

Index to Introductions and Annexes

Note: This index is provided as a general tool for accessing categories within the classifications and discussions of issues and key terms in the Introduction and Annexes.

Access, 14

Activities and Participation,
  component, 3, 7-10, 12-14, 20, 23,
  129-130

Activities and Participation List, uses of,
  248-251

Activities and Participation, structuring
  options, 248-251

Activity, activities, xv, xxi, 3, 7, 8, 10, 12,
  13, 14-8, 129, 229, 249-251, 265

Activity limitations, 3, 9, 12-4, 129, 228,
  249, 252-4

Actual environment, 249, 252-4

Adolescence, xv-xvi, vii, xii-xiii, 45, 107,
  129
  independence in ~, xv

Adolescents, see adolescence

Age specific, xv, 101

Aging, 266

Anatomical parts, 3, 8-11, 107, 228, 232,
  242

Anchor points, disability 20, 236

Architecture, 210

Assessment
  clinical ~, 5
  instruments, general ~, 15, 19, 20-21,
    45, 107, 130, 190, 237

Assessment instruments and ICF,
  236, 263

Assistive devices or personal assistance,
  xvii, 14-15, 23, 129, 170-171, 243-4

Attitudes, 15, 18, 189, 207-8, 229-230,
  246, 250, 253-4, 256

Attitudinal environment, 9, 15, 189, 246

Awareness, 5

Barrier, environmental, xx, 237, 252-3,
  256

Behaviour pattern, 15

Biomedical
  standards, 12
  status, 11

Body functions, 3-4, 8-12, 15, 17, 20, 23,
  45, 96-9, 227-8, 230-1, 233-5, 237-41,
  252, 265

Body functions, standard, 45, 240

Body organs, 10, 12

Body structure, 4, 7, 9-11, 20-21, 23, 35,
  68-70, 107, 228-9, 231-2, 234-5, 239-42

Body structures, standard, 107-8, 242

Body systems, 4, 7, 10, 45, 228, 240

Brain, functions of, 46-61

Capacity, construct of, 10, 230, 243, 249

Capacity, as qualifier, 13-14, 20, 237,
  243-5, 249-51

Capacity, as qualifier 'without assistance',
  243-4, 250

Case
  examples, 18, 252-4
  vignettes, xxii

Categories in ICF, 20, 227-30, 255

Causation, etiology, 13

Character style, 15

Child, vii-xxii
  -centered pedagogy, xiv
  in the context of the family, the, xv
  functioning ~'s, xv
  performance ~'s, xv

Childhood, xi, xii, xiii, xvi,
  early ~, xvi
  middle ~, xvi

Children, vii, viii, xi, xii, xiii, xiv, xv, xvi,
  xvii, xviii, xix, xxi, xxii, xxiii

Classification
  categories, 230-2
  components of ICF ~, 230
  granularity, 232
  levels, 232
  of dimensions of disability, xix
  parts of ICF ~, 232-5
  scope of ICF ~ 3, 7, 12
  unit of ICF ~, 7-8, 10, 20, 232
  universe of ~ in ICF, 7

Clinical applications of ICF 5, 280-263

Clinical use of ICF, ethical guidelines,
  257-8

Coding
  body functions, 107-8, 242
  body structures, 107-8, 242
  convention, code "8", 236-7, 241-3
  Environmental Factors, 189-90

evidence for ~, xxi

generic scale, 20

in ICF, 3, 5, 11, 12, 15, 21-3, 21-2, 23, 234-47

in ICF-CY, xix

options for Activities and Participation, 248-51

relevance to health condition, 238-9

Confidentiality, *See* Clinical use of ICF, ethical guideline

Consequence of disease, 4

Constructs in ICF, 3, 8, 17-8, 230-32

Contextual factors, 7, 8, 10-1, 15, 16, 243, 227, 246, 250, 260

Coping styles, 15

Cultural applicability and ICIDH, 261

Cultural organizations, 8, 262

Cultural variation and classification, 229, 260

Data comparability and ICF, 5

Decision-making, 4

Definitions
    in ICF, 236
    in classifications, 232

Determinants of health, 4

Developmental
    delay, xv
    stages, viii
    skills, xv

Diagnosis, 3, 4

Disability, xviii, 3, 4, 7, 8, 10, 11, 17, 18, 19-21, 241, 243, 246, 272
    as a medical issue, 19
    as a political issue, 19
    compensation systems, 5
    lived experience of ~, 13, 129, 243

Disabled Peoples' International, 255

Discrimination, social, 14, 18

Disease, 3, 4, 11-12, 13, 14, 18, 98, 165, 219, 228, 234, 259, 261, 264

Disease, consequence of, 4

Disfigurement, 18

Disorder, 4, 8, 12, 227-8

Domain, of disability, 3, 7, 8, 10, 13, 15, 20, 22, 227

Dutch Collaborating Centre for ICIDH, 260

Educational uses of ICF, 5

Education for All-World Education Forum, xiii

Environment
    actual ~, 13, 243, 245
    attitudinal ~, xvi, 8-9, 13, 15, 19
    current, 7, 10, 13, 18, 23, 129, 230, 243, 245, 252, 259, 260, 262, 268, 269, 271, 264
    social ~, xv, 14, 18, 255
    standard or uniform ~, 3, 11, 15, 20-1, 129, 215, 220, 222, 227-9, 237, 259, 241, 243, 245, 262, 261

Environmental
    factors, 189-90
    factor, barrier, xx, 237, 252-3, 256
    factor, facilitator, 6, 11, 17, 23, 189-90, 229, 232, 237, 243, 246-7, 256, 11, 17, 22, 24, 244, 252, 260, 262-3, 273
    modification, 5

Environmentally adjusted ability, 13, 129, 230, 243

Environments, xvi

Ethical guidelines for the use of ICF, 257-8

Event classification, 238

Exclusion terms in ICF, 236

Facilitator, environmental, 6, 11, 17, 22, 23, 189-90, 229, 244, 252, 260, 262, 263, 232, 237, 243, 246-7, 256

Field trials, during ICIDH-2 revision, 3, 261

French Collaborating Centre for ICIDH, 260

Functioning, xviii, 3, 4, 7, 8, 9-10, 11, 13-14, 15, 18, 17-21, 20, 21, 227, 238-9, 246-50, 253

Functioning, process of, 17

Gender, 7, 15, 228

Genetic abnormality, 12

Genetic predisposition, 15, 227

Geriatrics, 21, 35

Good life, 227

Habits, 15

Handicap, 3, 229, 255, 243, 272, 259-60

Health
    care systems, 5, 6
    care workers, 5
    components of ~, 4

condition, 3, 4, 7, 8, 12, 16, 17, 14-8,
    189, 217-8, 227-9, 238-9, 246, 253
condition, etiology of ~, 4, 2
determinants of ~, 4
domains, 3, 7, 22, 241-2, 227-8
information systems, 5, 265
insurance, 5
outcomes, 4, 5
outcome evaluation, 5, 23, 235
policies, 5
promotion, 6
-related domains, 3, 7, 227-8
research, 4, 5
states, 15, 16, 17, 20, 21, 227, 229, 235
statistics, 5
system, 229
Human rights, 6,

ICD-10, vii, xi, 3, 12, 228, 234
ICF
    aims of ~, 5
    and data comparability, 5
    applications, 5
    as a framework, 3, 4, 6, 7, 16, 264
    browser, 239
    case-recording forms, 264
    clinical use versions, 263
    computerization, 264
    constructs, 3, 8, 18, 17-8
    databases, 264
    definitions in ~, 263
    derived version of ~, vii
    exclusion terms in ~, 236
    full (detailed) version, 9, 11, 20, 263
    future directions for ~, 263
    inclusion terms in, 236
    minimal health information, 265
    operational definitions in, 20, 232,
        236, 263
    presentation of, 8
    properties of, 7-8
    research versions of, 280
    satisfaction or feeling of involvement
    or satisfaction, coding, 24
    short (concise) version, 8, 20, 263
    structural features of, 20
    training materials, 264
    use of ~, 20
ICF-CY

age range, xi
background, xi
development of ~, xii
activities, viii, xi
field trials, viii
history, xvii
issues relating to children and youth in
    the ~, xv
purpose of ~, xii
rationale, xi
    practical ~, xii
    philosophical, xiii
steps in using ~, xix
uses of ~, xvii
WHO Work Group, vii, viii, xvii
ICIDH
    1980, 5, 11, 12, 17
    revision, 259-60
Ideologies, 15
Impairment, 3-4, 8, 9-12, 11-13, 15, 16,
    17-21, 22, 24, 23, 45, 56, 63-5, 227-9,
    240
    identifying ~, 241
    scaling severity, 242
    interrelationship between ~, 241
Individual perspective on functioning and
    disability, 3, 7, 8, 10, 13, 14, 15, 16, 17,
    20, 243
Individual's health profile, coding, 238
Infancy, xv, xvi
Infants, xi
Information
    matrix, 13, 234-4, 249-50
    systems, 5, 265
Injury, 4, 8, 11, 14, 228, 254
International classifications, WHO family
    of, vii, 3, 4
International Organization for
    Standardization (ISO), 109, 264
Intervention matching, ICF use, 264
Involvement in a life situation, 9, 12, 13,
    129, 229, 242, 243, 248, 249

Law reform and ICF, 5, 6
Leprosy, 18
Life
    areas, 10, 12, 176-85
    events, 15
    experiences, 229

Life span, variations, 48, 233
Lifestyle, 15, 18
Lived experience of disability, 3, 129, 243

Managed health care, 6
Maturity
    psychological, xv
    physical, xv
    social, xv
Mental (or psychological) functions,
    9-11, 45, 228
Mental health, 35, 260, 263, 266, 267, 278,
    247, 250
Mental health applications of ICF, 250
Mental illness, 18
Mental retardation, 48
Model of disability, biopsychosocial, 19
ICF, 17
    interactive, 8, 17
    medical, 11, 18-9
    social, 18-9
Morbidity information, 4, 12
Mortality information, 4
Muscle atrophy, 18

National Center on Birth Defects and
    Developmental Disabilities of the
    Centers for Disease Control and
    Prevention, xvii
Neutral terms in the ICF, 233
North American Collaborating Centre for
    ICIDH, 260
Numeric coding in ICF, 10, 20, 235

Operational definitions in the ICF, 210,
    232, 236, 263, 264
'Other specified', use in ICF, 236

Participation, xv, xvi, xxi, 3, 6, 8, 10, 11,
    14, 15, 16, 18, 20, 243, 259, 264, 267
    restriction, 229
    standard, 243
Pathology, 11
People with disabilities, 5, 7
    ICF and ~, 252
Performance, as construct, 8, 10, 13-5,
    17-8, 19, 21, 23, 24, 230, 259-32, 265,
    267, 249
Performance, as qualifier, 14, 129, 243-4,
    250

Personal factors, 8, 9, 10, 15, 16, 17, 18,
    228-29, 230-31, 234, 260, 264
Physiological functions, 3, 9, 10, 45, 228
Planning, 5,
Population health, 4
Population health surveys, 6
Population studies and surveys, 5
Possible uses of the Activities and
    Participation list, 248
Poverty, 217-219
Practice Manual, xxii
Prevention, 6, 12, 219
Psychological assets, 16
Psychological functions, 9, 10, 11, 45

Qualifier, viii, xi, xv, xvi-xx, 8, 10, 12-4,
    20, 23, 237, 252
    body functions and structure, 45, 240
    body structure, 107-8, 242
    environmental factors, 189-90
    Activities and Participation, 129-30
    optional for activities and
        participation, 244-5, 249
    scaling, 242
Quality assurance, 5
Quality of life, 5, 264
Questionnaire application of ICF, 236

Race, 7, 15, 18
Reasons for contact with health
    services, 3
Rehabilitation services, xiv, 21, 219, 235,
    259, 263
Respect, *See* Ethical guidelines for use of
    ICF
Risk factors, 4
Rural or urban setting, 236

Salamanca Statement on the Right to
    Education, xiv
Sanitation of terms, 255
Service utilization, 13
Social
    action, 5
    background, 17
    benefit programmes, 264
    capital, 189, 246
    change, 18-9
    environment, xv, 9
    policy, 5

security, 5, 6
status, 175, 229
use of ICF information, ethical
    guidelines, 257-8
Societal perspective on disability, 7, 14,
    229
Socioeconomic characteristics, 7
Standard Rules for the Equalization of
    Opportunities, xiv
Standard Rules for the Equalization of
    Opportunities for Persons with
    Disabilities (1993), 5, 188
Stigma, 14, 18, 229, 253
Structure of ICF, 231, 232
Subjective well-being and ICF, 264
Suggested ICF data requirements for ideal
    and minimal health information
    systems or surveys, 265
Summary measures of population
    health, 4
Summary of the revision process, 259
Survey, application of ICF, 264
Symptoms and signs, 12

Task, 7, 9, 12, 13, 15, 140-4, 168-9, 242,
    266-7, 273
Taxonomic and terminological issues, 227
Taxonomic principles, 227

Terms, in the ICF, 3, 6, 7, 9, 12, 20, 189,
    227-30, 236, 248-50, 255, 263
Toddlers, xi
Trauma, 8, 18, 228

UNESCO, xvii
UNESCO's International Standard
    Classification of Education, 220
Uniform environment, 14, 243
United Nations, 5, 188, 277
United Nations Convention on the Rights
    of the Child, xi, xiii, xiv, 188
United Nations Convention on the Rights
    of Persons with Disabilities, xiii, xiv
United Nations Universal Declaration of
    Human Rights (1948), 188
Universalism and the ICF, 7
'Unspecified', use in ICF, 236

Values, 207, 249, 250

Well-being, 227-28, 264
WHO family of classifications., 260
World Health Assembly, 3, 24, 259,
    261-262

Youth, vii, viii, xi, xii, xiii, xiv, xv, xvi, xviii,
    xix, xxi

ICF-CY

Index to categories
within classifications

Note: This index is provided as a general tool for accessing categories within the classifications only. Only words actually found in the ICF-CY are indexed here with a reference to (a) code(s). When a reference to a word is on a higher level code in the classification, the same word can also appear in the more detailed classes underneath the higher level code. It is important to emphasize that index entries should not be used in any coding applications. For coding purposes, the full description of the code should be reviewed in the classification's applicable components. With use of the ICF-CY, a more comprehensive index may be developed that includes additional, extensive cross-references to the items found in the classification. Towards that end, WHO welcomes suggestions from users for terms and phrases that could be added to the index to increase its usefulness. For discussions of issues and key terms in the Introduction and Annexes in the original ICF, please refer to the Index in the main volume of the ICF.

Abdomen b28012, b5351
Abdominal b5250, b535
Abortions b660
Absence d6506
Absorption b515
Abstract b164, d1702, d1632, e465
Abstraction b164
Abuse d57022
Abused b130
Academic d810
Academics d9101
Acceptance d7102
Access d8300, d8250, d8200, d8150
Accessible e1502, e1501
Accessing d2305
Accommodation b215
Accomodating b1261
Accompanying b6403
Aching b280
Acids b5402
Acoustic b1560
Acquaintances d750, e425, e325
Acquire d1501
Acquiring d1502, d1501, d1500, d1452,
    d1451, d1450, d1402, d1401, d1400,
    d845, d815, d810, d155, d137, d134,
    d133, d132, d220, d210, d6
Act b1301, b640, b125
Acting b1641, d9202, d720, d2503
Acuity b210
Acute e5800, d2402
Adaptability b210, b125
Adaptation b21020, e215
Adaptations e1401, e1201
Adapting d2504, d2306
Adding d3501

Adjusting d4106, d540
Adopted d760, e5652
Adoption d7602
Adoptive d7600, e310
Adrenal s5803
Adult d8303, d8253, d8203, d7601,
    e57502, e57500
Advancing d845, d820
Aerobic b455
Aerophagia b510
Affect b152, e465, e160
Affection d3350
Affective b152
Agalactorrhoea b660
Age d7504, b7610, b4201, b4200, d475,
    e5752, e5751, e5750, e1450, e1200,
    e1152, e1150, e570, e325
Ageing e2150
Ageusia b250
Aggression d720
Agitation b147
Agreeableness b126
Aid e5552, e5551, e5550
Aids d6504, e1
Aircraft d4751, d470, e255
Airflow b440
Airway b4500
Airways b4501, b4500, b440
Akinetic b730
Alactation b660
Alcohol d57022
Alert b1102
Alertness b110
Algebra d1721
Allergic b435
Allergies b4351

Allocating b1642
Allodynia b2703
Allopathic e1101
Alone b21003, b21001, d9201, d855, d850, d163, d940
Alopecia b850
Alphabet d1451, d1400, d130
Alternating b7651
Altitude e210
Alveoli s43011
Ambitendency b147
Ambulance e5452, e5451, e5450
Amenorrhoea b650
Amicable b1261
Amino b5402
Amnesia b144
Amusement d920
Anabolism b540
Anaemia b430
Anaesthesia b2703, b265
Anal b525
Analgesia b2703, b280
Analysing b1646, d175
Anarthria b320
Anger b152
Animals d6404, d4503, d650, d480, d920, e220
Ankle b750, b710, s7502
Anopsia b2101
Anosmia b255
Antibody b435
Anticipating d5302
Antigens b4351
Antiques d9204
Antisocial b1267
Anuria b610
Anxiety b152
Anxiousness b1522
Apartment d610
Aphasia b167
Aphonia b310
Apnoea b440
Aponeuroses s7703
Appearance b860, b850, b750
Appetite b1302
Appliances d6301, d650, d640, d620, e1151, e1150
Appreciation d710
Apprenticeship d840

Apprenticeships e5853, e5850
Approachability b125
Approaching d2502
Appropriateness b152
Apraxia b176
Architecture e520, e515
Argument d3551, d3550
Arises b2403
Arising b670, b630, b535
Arithmetic b1721, d1502, d1500
Arm b7611, b7351, b7301, b760, s7300, d3350, d445
Arms b7603, d4550, d5401, d5400, d445, d430
Arousal b1522, b670, b640
Arrange d2303
Arranging d610, d2205, d2203, d2202, d2200, d2105, d2103, d2102, d2101, d2100
Arrhythmias b4101
Arterial b4150
Arteries b420, b415, s4101
Arteriosclerosis b415
Arthritis b710
Articular s7703
Articulation b340, b330, b320, b310
Artistic e1401, e585
Arts d920
Ascertaining b114
Ask d2402
Asking d3500, d730, d132
Asleep b1342
Aspiration b510
Assertive b1266
Asserts d310
Assets e2201, e350, e165
Assignment d2105, d2101
Assimilation b540, b530, b525, b520, b515
Assist e11521, e1552, e1502, e1251, e1201, e1151
Assistance e575, e570, e3
Assistant e340
Assistants e575, e440, e340, e310
Assisted e1550, e1500
Assisting d6
Assistive e5802, e5801, e1
Association d950 e5900, e345
Assuming d1631
Assure e1553, e1503

Astigmatism b210
Asymmetric b770
Ataxic b320
Atherosclerosis b415
Athethotic b7650
Athetosis b765
Atmospheric e230, e225
Atria s41000
Attachment b122
Attaining b560
Attending d8301, d8251, d8151, d1601,
 d1600, d855, d850, d820, d930
Attention b172, b167, b156, b147, b144,
 b140, b134, b114, d3350, d660, d161,
 d160
Attraction d7700
Audio e1551, e1501, e1250
Audiologists e355
Auditory b230, b156, s2603, d115, e2500,
 e1251, e1250
Aural b240
Authoritative e5855, e5854, e5852, e5851
Authorities e5
Authority d740, e5951, e5500, e430, e335,
 e330
Autobiographical b1441
Autoimmunity b435
Automatic b750, b620
Automatically b750
Automobile d4751
Automobiles d6503
Autonomy d940
Autumn e2255
Auxological b560
Avoid d4503
Avoiding d571, d570
Awakening d2302
Aware b1800, b1102, d7204, d5702,
 d5701, d5700, d331
Awareness b1644, b1442, b1144, b1143,
 b1142, b1141, b1140, b180, b110
Axillary s8402
Azoospermia b660

Babbling d331, b340, b310
Baby d470
Back b28013, b5102, s8105, d4107, d4105,
 d480, d430, e2450
Backache b28013
Background e2501

Backgrounds d750
Backpack d4703
Backwards d450
Balance b755, b555, b545, b540, b235
Balcony d4600
Ball d4455, d4454, d435
Banging d131, e250
Barking e2501
Bartering d860
Basal b540, s1103
Basic b5400, b163, b147, b117
Basis d8502, d8501, e5800, e340
Bath d5101
Bathing d6600, d510
Bathrooms d6402
Beat b460, b410
Beating b4101
Bed d4150, d420, d410, d2104, d2100
Bedsores b810
Behaviour b1644, d7102,
 b1471, b1470, d135, d130, d250
Behavioural b1470, b125
Behaviours b164, d720, d5602, d5601,
 d2306, d2303, e465
Believe d1630, d2105, d2101
Belonging d6101
Bench d420
Bend d4453
Bending d4553, d410
Benefit e165
Biceps b750
Bicycle d475, d435
Bile b515
Binaural b2301
Binocular b210
Biological b810
Birth d7602, e2150, e310
Biting d1203, b510
Bladder b630, b620, b610, s570, s6102,
 e1151
Bleeding b650
Blending b2301
Blindness b210
Bloated b535
Block b160, d1314
Blockage b415
Blocks d2102, d131, e11520
Blood b5152, b4
Blowing b450
Bodies e5855, e5854, e5852, e5851, e5351,
 e5101, e210

Boiling d6300
Bold b1266
Bone b720, b430, s4204
Bones b7, s75020, s75010, s75000, s73020,
    s73010, s73000, s7700, s7400, s7200,
    s7102, s7101, s7100
Books d4402, d166, e1451, e1300
Bottles d560, d550
Bowels e1151
Bowing d4105
Bowling d9201
Box d1312, d430
Bradycardia b410
Bradylalia b330
Bradypnoea b4400
Braille d3601, d325, d166, d145, d140,
    e5600, e1552, e1502, e1451
Brailler d1450
Brain b1, s110
Brainstorming d163
Branches e5951
Breakdown b540, b515
Breakfast d2302
Breaking d550
Breast b55501, s6302, d560, e110
Breath b4551, b460
Breathing b4402, b4401, b450, b445,
    d3100, e1151
Breaths b4400
Breeze e2254
Broadcast b1603
Broca b167
Bronchial b440, s43010
Brooms d640
Brotherly d7602
Bruising b820
Brush d4453, d1450
Brushes d640
Brushing d5201
Bruxism b7652
Budgeting d230
Building d4500, d1551, d460, d2104,
    d2102, d2100, e5200, e5152, e5151,
    e5150, e155, e150
Buildings d460, e515, e260, e255, e155,
    e150, e120
Burning b840, b280, b270, b220, d6405
Burping b510
Bursae s7703

Buses e1200
Business d8500, d865
Buying d865, d610
Buzzing e250

Cachexia b530
Calcium b545
Calculating d172
Calculation b1, d1721, d1720
Calculus d1721
Calling d360
Callosum s11070
Callus b810
Calluses d5200
Calm b1263
Canal s63033, s2501
Canals s2602
Canes d6504, e1201
Capillaries b415, s4103
Captioning e5600
Car d4200, d1314, d475, d470
Carbohydrate b540
Carbohydrates b540
Carbon b5401
Cardiac b4102
Cardiomyopathy b410
Cardiovascular b4, s4
Cards d9200, d2103, e1451
Care d7601, d815, d660, d650, d240, d5,
    e5855, e5854, e5852, e5851, e5802,
    e5801, e5800, e1500, e575, e440, e345,
    e340, e310
Caregiver b1403, d5702, d5602, d5601
Caregivers d57021, e340
Caring d6, d5
Carpal b720
Carriage b430, d4752, d470
Carry b4302, b4301, d240
Carrying b430, b164, d5602, d5601, d550,
    d540, d530, d8, d7, d6, d4, d3, d2
Cars d131, e11521, e1201, e1200
Carts d6503
Casual d9205, d750, d355, d350
Catabolism b540
Catatonia b147
Catch b2152
Catching d445
Categorization b164
Categorized e4

Cats e350
Cauda s12003
Cause b130, e230
Caused e2150, e255, e235
Cavity b5105
Celebrations d816
Cell b435, e2200
Cellulose e2200
Central b210
Centre d410, e57502
Cerebellum s1104
Ceremonies d9300, d910
Certificates d830
Cervical s76000, s12000
Cervix s63011
Cessation b6702
Chair d4350, d420, d410
Change e245, e215
Changes b5501, b4202, b1102, b555,
    b134, d4403, d3100, d1601, d2304, e2
Changing b1643, d4
Chanting b340, d930
Character b1471, b1102, d1451, d1450
Characterizing b125
Characters d1451, d166, d140
Charity d855
Cheeks b5100
Cheerful b1265
Chemical b810
Chess d1551, d9200
Chest b28011, b460
Chewing b510, d1203
Child b6603, b1403, d6605, d940, d3503,
    d815, d760, d430, d315, e1500, e575,
    e165
Childbirth b660
Children e1150, e310, e165
Chloroplasts e2200
Choice d177
Choking b460
Chop d4402
Chorea b765
Choreatic b7650
Choroid s2200
Church d4152, d930
Circadian b1340
Circuit b410
Circulation b410
Citizen d950

Citizenship d950, d940, d920, d910
City d6601, d4602
Civil e5500, e545, e530
Clarity b110
Claudication b4150
Clean d5101, d5100
Cleaning d5205, d5204, d5203, d530,
    d510, d6, e1150
Clearing b5105
Climate e225
Climatic d540
Clinics e5802, e5801, e5800
Clitoral b640
Clitoris s63030
Clothes d650, d640, d540, d240, e1150
Clothing d4403, d5301, d5300, d540, d6,
    e1651
Clotting b430
Clouding b1100
Clumsiness b760, b147
Cluttering b330
Coagulation b4303
Coccyx s76004
Cochlea s2600
Cochlear e1251
Cognitive b176, b172, b167, b164, b163,
    b160, b147, b144, b117, d815
Coherence b1601
Cold b5501, b2700, d630, d5700, d2200,
    e2250
Colleagues d7201, e425, e325
Collecting d9204, d640
Colleges d830
Coloration b850
Colouring d4402
Colour b1561, b210, e240
Colours b21021
Column s7600
Coma b110
Comfort d570
Comfortable d5700
Command d870
Commercial e5650, e5300, e5200, e5152,
    e5151, e5150, e555
Communal d9103
Communicable d5702
Communicating d660, d3, e5602, e5601
Communication e5100, e560, e535,
    e125, e115

Communities e5302, e595

Community d4601, d855, d815, d810, d750, e325

Comparing d6200

Compensation e5700

Competence d150, d145, d140, d137, d134, d133

Competencies d155

Competitive d9201, e5902, e5901

Completing d8252, d8152, d830, d820, d230, d220, d210

Complying d7203

Composition e2150

Compositions d1702, d1701

Comprehending d1661, d325, d320, d315, d310

Comprehension d166

Compulsions b160

Computations d172

Computer e5602, e5601, e5600, e5352, e5351, e5350, e1351, e1301, e1300, e1251

Computers d3601, d3600

Computing b1720, d172

Concentration b140

Concept b1344, b164, d1501

Concepts d1720, d1501, d163, d137, d132

Conceptualized b1602

Condition e5752, e5751, e5750, e570

Conditioning e2600

Condoms d570

Conduction b167

Confidence b126

Conflict e235

Conflicting b1646

Congruence b1520

Conjunction d2

Conjunctiva s2200

Connection b3300, d930

Conscientiousness b126

Conscious b1301

Conservation d6404, e5202, e5201, e5200, e160

Consistency b525

Consolidated b1440

Constipation b525

Constituents b4300

Constitutional b126, e5952, e5951

Constriction b780, b415

Construction e520, e515, e155, e150

Consume b1303

Consumer e5301, e510

Consumers e5300

Consuming d5701, d560, d550

Consumption b5400, e565, e110

Contact d3500, d710, d5602, d5601, e1251

Contacting d845

Containing e2200

Continence b620, b525

Contour b2100

Contract d8500

Contracted d8500

Contraction b7801, b7651, b5250, b750, b740, b730, b410

Contractions b7502, b7501, b7500, b5352, b765, b755

Control b6202, b5253, b1521, b770, b765, b760, b710, b160, b147, b130, d4402, d940, d475, d240, e11521, e1351, e1151, e5

Controlling d4155, d720

Conventions d1701, d720, d5404, e5

Conversation d350-d369

Conversing d350

Conversion b540

Convey d335, d170, d145

Conveying d3352, d3351, d3350, d340

Cooing b3401

Cooking d6502, d640, d630, d620

Cooling b830

Cooperation b2152

Cooperative b1261, d8803

Coordinate d1551

Coordinated d446, d445, d440, d435, d550, d540, d250, d240, d230, d220, d210

Coordinating b1641, d5302, d5301, d5300

Coordination b1471, b760, b3100

Cope d2402, d2401

Coprolalia b7652

Copying d130

Cord s120

Cornea s2201

Corns d5200

Coronary b410

Corporations e5650

Corpus s11070

Corridors e1552, e1502
Cortical s1100
Cosmetics d5200
Coughing b450
Counting d1501, d135
Cousins d760
Crafts d8500, d810, d920
Cramp b5352
Cramps b535
Cranial s1106
Cranium s7100
Craving b130
Crawling b840, d460, d455
Create d465, e465
Creating b1640, d7504, d7503, d7502,
    d7501, d7500, d770, d760, d740, d163,
    e5200
Creation d865, e5902, e5901, e5102,
    e5101, e5100
Creed e325
Criminal e5500
Crises d240
Crisis d240
Criticism d710
Cross d4153, d4103
Crouched d4101
Crowded d4503
Crushing b5102
Crutches e1201
Crying b340
Cues d1660, d710
Cultural d9202, e5552, e5551, e5550,
    e330, e140
Culture d6301, d5404, d920, e1152, e460,
    e315, e310, e140
Cup d1312, d430
Curbs d4551
Curious b1264
Curricula e5855, e5854, e5852, e5851
Curriculum d845, d830, d825, d820
Customary d3502, d3500, e5502, e5501
Cutting b5101, d6300, d4402, d550
Cycle b6702, b6701, b650, b134
Cycles b6501, e245
Cyclical b555

Daily d640, d620, d325, d230, e115
Dancing d9202
Danger d2402, d2306

Day d815, d2200, d230, e57501, e335,
    e245, e235
Deafness b230
Death e2150
Debate d355
Deceitful b1267
Deciding b164, d2402, d177
Deciphering d1400
Decision b164, e330
Decisions d220, d210, d1
Decisive d2402
Declaration d940
Decoding b1670
Decorating d6102
Decrease b1470, b540
Decreased b1344, b515, b420
Decryption b167
Defecation b535, b525, b520, b515, d530
Defensive b755
Deferred d135
Defiant b1261
Deficiency b545
Defining d137
Dehydration b545
Delayed b660, b640
Delirium b110
Delivering e5800, e5700
Delivery e5855, e5854, e5852, e5851,
    e5302
Delusions b160
Demand b1251
Demanding d240
Dementia b117
Demographic e325, e215
Demonstrative b1260
Dental d5201
Dentition s32001, s32000
Depart d2305
Dependable b1267
Dependent b164, e165
Depersonalization b1800
Derealization b1800
Derive e5951
Dermatome b280
Design e520, e515, e160, e155, e150
Designation e1552, e1502
Designed d4702, d815, d465, e5, e1
Designers e360
Designs d3152

Desire b1302
Desk d4452, d4153
Desks e1351
Despairing b1265
Destination d6601
Destruction e235
Detected b1564, b1563
Detection b2300
Determination b2352, b172, d940, e5252
Determined d4155, e2601, e2600, e2501, e2500
Determining b2352, b2351, b2350, b2304, b2303, b2302, e5700, e5401
Develop b122
Developing b1641, d175, d155, d150, d145, d140, d137, d134, d133, e5252
Developmental b530, b125
Device d4703, d1450
Devices e5802, e5801, e1401, e1251, e1250, e1201, e1151
Dial d440
Dialogue d3504, d3503, d3502, d3501, d3500
Diaphragm b445, s43031
Diarrhoea b525
Diastolic b4201, b4200
Dictate e5855, e5852
Diencephalon s1102
Diet b5403, b5402, b5401, d570
Differentiating b21021, d7106
Differentiation b2301, d7106
Differing e2201
Difficulty b122, d2402
Dilation b4152, b4150
Dining d550
Dinner d2204
Dioxide b5401
Diplopia b210
Directed b7602, b1472, b164, b160
Directing d161
Direction b5107, b5106, b2352, d475
Directions b2152, d3352, d820, d730
Disabilities d940
Disability e5752, e5751, e5750, e570
Disagreement d7103, d335
Disasters e5302, e235
Discharge b650, b620
Discomfort b6702, b6701, b6700
Discriminating b1645, b1561, b1560, b230

Discrimination b230, d950
Discussing d3503
Discussion d3504, d3502, d355
Discussions d3504
Disease b7356, e5800
Diseases d5702
Disengagement b134
Dishes d6401, d6301
Dislocation b715
Disorders b7650
Disorientation b114
Displaying d172
Disposal d6405, d475
Disposing d640
Disposition b126, b125
Dispositions b126, b125
Dispute d175
Disruptable b1440
Disruption b1470, e235, e230
Dissatisfaction b6403
Dissemination e5602, e5601
Dissociative b144
Distances d4602, d450
Distension b5351
Distinct b1640, b126, b125
Distinguishing b2304, b1565, b1564, b1563, b1562
Distortion b21023
Distractibility b140
Distracting d160, e260, e250, e240
Distraction d240
Distractions e2601, e2600, e2501, e2401
Distributing e5700
Distribution e5902, e5901, e5602, e5601, e565
Disturbance e255
Disturbances e235
Diurnal b1340
Diversion d920
Dividing b140, d172
Diving d4553
Division b1720
Dizziness b240
Doll d1314, d1313
Dolorosa b2703
Domestic d855, d6
Domesticated e350, e220
Dominance b147
Door d4401, d445, e2401, e1550, e1500
Doors e1550, e1500, e1351

Downhearted b1265
Drafting d170
Drawing b5100, d660, d335, d130, e1251
Dreaming b1344
Dress d5404
Dressing b176, d6600, d1313, d2200, d5
Dribbling b620
Drink b5153, b5152, b5105, b1302, d630,
    d620, d560, e110
Drinking b535, d4301, d630, d5
Driven d470
Driving b1301, d480, d475, d470, d465,
    d240, e4
Drooling b510
Dropping d4403, d1310
Drug b110, d5702
Drug-induced b1102
Drugs d57022, e110
Drying d640, d5
Ducts b2153, s570
Dull b280
Dusting d6402
Duties d8301, d8251, d8201, d8151,
    d2400, d950, d230
Dwarfism b560
Dwelling d7503, d650, d610, e155
Dwellings d7501, e525
Dynamics b410
Dysarthria b320
Dysdiadochokinesia b760
Dysfluency b3300
Dysfunction b7650
Dysfunctions b430
Dyskinesia b765
Dysmenorrhoea b670
Dyspareunia b670
Dysphagia b510
Dysphonia b310
Dyspnoea b460
Dystonias b7356, b7350
Dystonic b765

Ear b240, b235, s2
Ears b240
Eat d6604
Eating b535, d6600, d6401, d1550, d630,
    d2302, d5
Echolalia b147
Echopraxia b147

Economic e5951, e590, e570, e565, e330,
    e165
Economical d870
Economy e5902, e5901
Ectopic pregnancy b660
Edible d630
Education d8, e5100, e1152, e590, e585,
    e340, e130
Educational d8203, d8202, d8201, d8200,
    d830, d815, e1300
Effacing b1266
Effect b1102
Effectively d145
Effects d177, d175
Effort b1254, d2503
Ejaculation b640
Elbow b710, s73001
Elbows b7603
Elderly d7601, d6605
Elected e5950
Election e5952
Elections e595
Electricity e530, e240
Electrolyte b555, b545, b540
Electrolytes b545
Electromagnetic e240
Electronic e5352, e5351, e5350, e1551
Elementary d1550, d1501, d1500, d1452,
    d1451, d1450, d1402, d1401, d1400
Elevators e1501
Eligibility e5855, e5854, e5852, e5851,
    e5802, e5801, e5752, e5751, e5702,
    e5701, e5700, e5401, e5352, e5252
Elimination b5, d530
Emaciation b530
Email d3600
Embracing d3350
Embryos e2200
Emergencies d2401
Emergency e5452, e5451, e5450, e5300,
    e1553, e1503
Emotion b152
Emotional b152, b130, b126, b125, d7700,
    d7600
Emotionally b1264
Emotions d720, d2504, d2503, d2502,
    d2501, d2500
Emphysema b440
Employed d850, e590

Employee d7401, d850
Employer d7400
Employers d845, d740, e330
Employing d1700
Employment d910, d660, d650, e5652,
    e5651, e5650, e5100, e590, e135
Enabling e540
Enact d1314
Ending d7201, d355, d350
Endurance b740, b735, b730, b455
Energy b540, d2504, d2303, e5300, e2500,
    e2400
Engagement d920, d880
Engaging b6401, d1630, d8802, d865,
    d860, d855, d850, d840, d835, d830,
    d825, d820, d816, d730, d2300, d950,
    d930, d920, d910
Enjoying d950, d940
Enjoyment d920
Ensure d870, d5700
Ensuring d6605, d650, d570
Enter d8303, d8253, d8203,
    d8153
Entering d750, e1550, e1500, e1451
Entitlements d870
Entrances e155, e150
Entries e1550, e1500
Entry e1550, e1500, e1351
Enunciation b320
Environment b2401, b1565, b1142, b180,
    b134
Environmental b5501
Enzyme b515
Equalization d940
Equals d740
Equilibrium b5452, b5451
Equina s12003
Equipment d865, d475, d470, d465,
    d2205, e5802, e5801, e255, e1
Equipping d6102
Erection b640
Ergonomics e5900
Errands d2201
Erratic b1263, b1253
Escalators e1501
Esophageal b5106
Establish b122
Establishing d7200, d930
Establishment e5552, e5551

Estate e5250
Esteem d7500, d710
Ethics d9100
Ethnicity e325
Etiquette e465
Eukaryotic e2200
Eustachian s2501
Evaluating b1645, d177, d175
Evaluation d8302, d8252, d8202, d8152
Exam d8302, d8252, d8202
Examination d355
Examinations d570
Exams d240
Exchange b440, d6201, d6200, d6101,
    d3503, d865, e535, e165
Exchanging d860
Excitement b6400, b147
Excretion b5452, b5451
Excretory b620, b610
Excursions d816
Executive b164, e5951
Exercise b740, b4
Exercising d6506
Exert d4402, d4350
Exertion b455
Exhaling b440
Exit e1550, e1500, e1351
Exiting e1550, e1500
Exits e155, e150
Expectations d2504, d2503, d2501
Expelling b5107
Experience b1522, b1521, b180, b140,
    b126
Experiences b1802, b1250, b163, d250,
    d110-d129
Exploring d1203, d1202, d1201, d1200
Expressing d3500, d330
Expression b167, b126, b125, d310,
    d2504, d2503, d2502, d2501, d2500,
    d130
Expressions d3502, d3150
Expressive b167
Expulsion b5254
Extend d4452
Extended d760, e415, e340, e315, e310
Extending d4553
External b7502, b215, b140, s6303, s3100,
    s2303, s240
Exteroceptive b750

Extramuscular s7703
Extraversion b126
Extremities d435
Extremity s8104, s8102, s750, s730
Eye b21003, b21002, b21001, b21000,
    b1474, b1471, b1344, b760, b730, b220,
    b215, s2, d3500, d5602, d5601
Eyeball s220
Eyebrow s2302
Eyelid b215, s2301
Eyes b21002, b21000, b2152, d315

Face s7101, d4150, d1600, d520, d510,
    e1250
Facial s8401, d3350, d3150, d130
Facilitate b215, d465, e135
Facilitating e1351, e1151
Facilities e5802, e5801, e5800, e5500,
    e155, e150
Factual e4
Faecal b525
Faeces b525
Failure b410
Fall b4201
Falling b240, e2253
Fallopian s63012
Falls d4403
Familiar d7106, e325
Family d2204, d810, d9, d7, e57501,
    e57500, e415, e410, e340, e335, e315,
    e310
Farm e2201, e1600
Fasciae s75023, s75013, s75003, s73023,
    s73013, s73003, s7703, s7602, s7403,
    s7203, s7105
Fast b4400, b4100
Fasteners d6500
Fat b1801, b540
Fatiguability b455
Fatigue b4552
Fats b540
Fauna e220
Fear b152
Feasting d550
Feeding d1313, d650, d560
Feeling b1801, b630, b535, b280, b265,
    b152, d5700, d120
Feelings b1522, b460, b220, d710, d134,
    d133
Feet b28015, b7603, d4556, d4552, d4153,
    d4103, d435, b730, b710, d510

Female b660
Fertility b660
Fertilizing d6505
Figure b21022
Figures d1400
Filing e1351
Filling d4402
Filtering d160
Filtration b610
Financial e5650, e165
Find e5900, e1552, e1502
Finding d7200, d845, d2304, d175, d172,
    d930, e1552, e1502, e590
Finger b7611, s8300, d520
Fingernails d5203
Fingers s73021, d4455, d4454, d4453,
    d4451, d4450, d1201, d5203, d440
Finishing d3502, d240
Fire d315, d571, e5452, e5451, e5450,
    e5152, e5151
Fitness d920, d570
Fixation b2101, b215
Fixing d650
Flaccid b320
Flattening b152
Flatulence b525
Flexibility b164
Flight b160
Floor s620, d4600, d4556, d4555, d4153,
    d4151, d4101, e1552, e1502
Flora e220
Flossing d5201
Fluency b761, b340, b330, d140
Fluids b650
Flushes b6702
Focusing b140, d160
Folding d640
Folds s3400
Fontanelle s71001
Food b4351, b1302, b525, b515, b510,
    d4403, d1203, d860, d2204, d550, d6,
    e1651, e110
Foot b760, s7502, d4553, d4350, d4106,
    d450, d446
Footwear d6500, d640, d540
Force b5100, b1301, b730, b410, d4454,
    d4350
Forearm s7301

Formally d9201
Formation b820, b810, b164, b122
Formulating d163
Fossae s3102
Foster d760, e310
Freedoms d950
Friend d3503, d360, d345, d2201
Friends d9205, d7, e57500, e420, e340, e320
Friendship d7500
Friendships d7200
Frigidity b640
Frontal b164, s11000
Frowning d3350
Fugue b1101
Fulfilling d8301, d8251, d8201, d8151, d2302
Funding e5802, e5801
Furnishing d610
Furniture d6102, d650, d2105, d2101, e1150

Gagging b460
Gait b1471, b770, b765, b760
Galactorrhoea b660
Gall s570
Games d3504, d2103, d155, d920, d880, e11520
Gametes b6600
Ganglia s1103
Gardening d6505
Garments d640
Gas b535, e2600
Gases b5254, b440
Gastro b5106
Gastrointestinal b5352, b515
Gather d6201
Gathering d620
Gatherings d9205, d9103, e465
Gaze b2101
Gender e325
Genital b640-b679
Genitalia s6303
Genitals b6703, d520
Geometry d1721
Gestural b16713, b16703
Gesture d130
Gestures b16713, b16703, d335, d315, d135

Gesturing b1470
Gigantism b560
Give d3352, d3101
Giving d7104, d845, d2204
Gland b555, b550, b545, b530, s5803, s5802, s5801, s5800, s2300
Glands b4353, b215, b5, s820, s580, s510
Glandular b830
Glans s63050
Glass d4301, d4300
Glasses e1251
Globus b535
Gloomy b1265
Gloves d540
Glucose b5401
Gluten b5153
Goal b1472, b164, b160, d8803, d163
Goal-directed b160
Going d920
Goods d860, d650, d640, d630, d620, d610, e165, e5
Government e5951, e5252
Governmental d950
Grammar d145
Grammatical b1672, d1701
Grandparents d7603, e310
Grapheme d1451
Graphic d3152, d1330
Graphs d3152
Grasp d4455, d4452, d1402
Grasping d1661, d440
Gravel d4502
Gravis b740
Gravity d410
Greetings d3500
Grinding b5102
Grip b2402
Grooming d650
Ground b21022, b2301, d4556, d4554, d4553, d4552, d4305, d450, e1200
Group b7801, b765, d3504, d9202, d9201, d855, d332, d240, d220, d210, e1152, e460, e335
Groups b780, b740, b735, b730, d9101, d9100, d855, d850, e555, e215
Growing d6505, d3152
Growth b860, b850, b117, b5, e2201
Guardians d760, e330
Guardrails e1553, e1503

Guessing d1631
Guidance d2300
Gums s3201
Gurgling b3401
Gustatory b250, b156
Gymnastics d9201

Haematological b545, b4
Haemophilia b430
Hair b55500, s840, d520, d510
Hallucination b156
Hand b1473, b1471, b1470, b760, s7302,
    d6400, d3350, d3150, d445, d440
Handicrafts d9203
Handles d445, e1550, e1500
Handling d430-d449, d2
Hands b28014, b16713, b16712,
    b16703, b16702, b7603, b730, b710,
    d4550, d4403, d4402, d4401, d4400,
    d1201, d445, d430, d510
Handwriting e1251
Hanging d6400
Happiness b152
Hardening b810
Harm d571
Harms d570
Harshness b3101, e2501
Harvesting d6201
Hate b152
Haunches d4101
Hazardous d571, e1553
Head b28010, b7653, s8100, s710, d4155,
    d5401, d5400, d5202, d430, d335
Headgear d5401, d5400
Healing b820
Health d6506, d815, d660, d5
Healthy e580
Heard e250
Hearing d115, e5500, e1251
Heart b4, s4100
Heat b5501, b2700, d630, e2250
Heating d6300
Heavy d240
Height d3152, e2252
Help d2402, e340
Helping d6606, d6604, d6603, d6602,
    d6600, d6507, d6406, d6302
Hemianopia b210
Hemiparesis b7401, b7352, b7302

Hemiplegia b7401, b7352, b730
Hemiplegic b770
Herbs e1100
Heritage e5202, e5201
Hide d9200, d2103
Hip b28016, b715, b710, s75001, d430
Hired d845
Hissing b2400
Hitting d131
Hoarseness b310
Hobbies d920
Home d6601, d2305, d2302, d2204, d855,
    d815, d810, d460, e57501, e5802,
    e5801, e5800, e155, e3
Homeless e5250
Hopeful b1265
Hopping d4553
Hormonal b555
Hospitals e5802, e5801, e5800
Hot b6702, d5700
House d7503, d660, d650, d640, d610,
    d460, e5150
Housekeeping d6504
Houses e5250, e1651, e1450
Housework d650, d640, d630, e5100, e575
Housing e525
Human d3100, d1600, d475, d470, d115,
    d950, d940, d530, e5900, e4, e2, e1
Humanity d940
Humans d4703, e235
Humidity e2601, e2600, e225
Humming b340
Hunger b460
Husband d770
Hydramnios b660
Hydration d5200
Hydrography e210
Hydronephrosis b610
Hygiene d5205, d5201
Hypaesthesia b2702
Hypalgesia b2703
Hyperacidity b515
Hyperadrenalism b555
Hyperaesthesia b2702, b265
Hyperalgesia b280
Hypercalcaemia b545
Hypergonadism b555
Hyperkalaemia b545
Hypermenorrhoea b6502

Hypermetropia b210
Hypermobility b710
Hypermotility b515
Hypernasality b310
Hypernatraemia b545
Hyperparathyroidism b555
Hyperpathia b2703
Hyperpituitarism b555
Hypersensitivities b5153, b4351
Hypersensitivity b21020, b435
Hypersomnia b134
Hypertension b420
Hyperthermia b550
Hyperthyroidism b5400, b555
Hypertonia b735
Hyperventilation b440
Hypoadrenalism b555
Hypocalcaemia b545
Hypogeusia b250
Hypogonadism b555
Hypokalaemia b545
Hypomenorrhoea b6502
Hyponasality b310
Hyponatraemia b545
Hypoparathyroidism b555
Hypopituitarism b555
Hyposensitivity b21020
Hyposmia b255
Hypotension b420
Hypothermia b550
Hypothesizing d1632
Hypothyroidism b5400, b555
Hypotonia b735
Hypotonic b610

Icons d3351, d3151, d1400, d166
Ideas b1672, b164, b160, d1452, d350,
    d170, d163
Ideation b176
Ideational b160
Identifying b1646, d175
Ideomotor b176
Idiomatic d310
Ill d5702
Illusion b156
Image b180
Images d163, e2401
Imaginary d1630
Imaginative b1264

Imitating d331, d130
Imitation d135, d130
Immobile d4503
Immune b435, s420
Immunization b435
Immunizations d570
Impaired b210
Implants e1251
Implementing d177, e5901, e5801, e5651,
    e5501, e5251, e5151
Implements d1450, d550
Impotence b640
Impulse b130
Impulses d720
Inaction b1252
Inattentive b1264
Incentive b1301
Incoherence b160
Income e570
Incompetence b525
Incomplete b630, d1631
Incongruent b1646
Incontinence b620, b525
Independently d720, d220, d210
Indicate d335
Indicates d3152
Indicating b280, d570, d560, d550, d530
Individual b761, b130, b126, b125, e345,
    e255, e230, e4, e1
Individuals b1142, d7106, d770, e2150,
    e1602, e1151, e460, e345, e340, e335,
    e330, e325, e320, e315, e310, e5
Indoor d650, e5400, e260, e155, e150,
    e120, e115
Induced b755, b750, b110
Industrial e5152, e5151, e5150
Inexpressive b1264
Infant b761
Infections b435
Influence e330, e4
Influenced e335
Information e5602, e5601, e535, e260,
    e250, e240, e125
Infrastructure e235
Ingestion e110, b5
Ingredients d630
Inhabitants d750
Inhaling b440
Inhibited b1260

Initiate d6603, d155
Initiating b1255, d71040, d3551, d3550,
    d3504, d3503, d3500, d2502, d2203,
    d2202, d2200, d210
Initiation d9102
Injury b4303, d5702, d571
Inquisitive b1264
Insecure b1266
Insight b164
Insomnia b134
Instances b1640
Institutional d810
Institutions e5853, e5850
Instructing d6201, d6200
Instruction d815
Instructions d3102, d166
Instrument d9202
Instruments d2103, d920, e1650
Insufficiency b610, b410
Insufficient b4152, b510
Insulating b810
Insurance e5702, e5701, e5700, e5650
Intake b5452, b5451
Intangible e165
Integrate b122, b117
Integrated d155, d220
Integrating b1646
Integrative b167
Integrity b715
Intellectual b160, b147, b144, b126, b125,
    b117, d7600, e1652
Intensity b21020, d1601, e250, e240
Intent d325
Interacting d8301, d8251, d8201, d8151,
    d720, d710
Interactions b122, d6603, d5602, d5601,
    d2502, d7
Interchange d350
Intercostal s43030
Intercourse b6401, b670
Interest b640, d7504
Interests d7500, d9100, e555, e325
Interior d6501
Intermediate d6201, d6200
Intermittent b4150
Internal b215, b140, s2603
Internet e5350, e560
Internship d840
Interpersonal d660, d7, e4
Interpretation d166

Interpreting b156
Interrelated d1751
Interval b650
Interventions e5800
Interview d8450
Intestinal b515
Intestine s540
Intestines b5254, b515
Intimate d7201, d7200, d770
Intolerance b515
Intonation b330
Introduce d815
Introducing d7200, d3501, d3500
Introversion b126
Inviting d2205
Involuntary b7801, b770, b765, b760,
    b755, b750
Involvement e5252
Involves b1470, d865
Iris b2150, s2202
Iron b545
Ironing d6500, d640
Irresponsible b1262
Irritable b1263
Irritation b240, b220
Isced e585
Ischaemia b4103
Isolated b7600, b7300, b740, b735
Itching b2404, b840, b220

Jerky e255
Job d855, d850, d845, d825, e5900
Jogging d455
Joining d8803, d8802, d8801
Joint b7651, b750, b715, b710, s75021,
    s75011, s75001, s73011, s73001
Joints b28016, b7, s75021, s73021, s7701,
    s7401, s7201, s7103
Joy b152
Judgement b164
Jumping d455
Jumps b2152
Justice e5502, e5501

Keep d8451
Keeping b54500, d6404, d845, d2401,
    d570, d540
Keloid b820
Keyboard d1450
Kicking b7611, d435

Kidney s6100
Kidneys b6100
Kilometre d4501, d4500
Kinaesthesia b260
Kinship d760
Kitchen e1551
Kneading d6301
Knee b710, s75011
Kneeling d415, d410
Knees b7603, d4550, d4152, d4102, d4101
Knife d4402
Knitting d9203
Knob d440
Knowing b163, b114
Knowledge b163, d1, e1652, e585, e130
Knows d7502, d355, d350

Labia s63032, s63031
Lability b152
Labour e5652, e5651, e5650, e1652,
    e1651, e1650, e590
Labyrinth s2601
Lachrymal b215, s2300
Lactation b660
Language b230, b340, b330, b320, b310,
    b1, d815, d170, d166, d134, d133, d3
Languages b16712, b16702
Larynx b310, s340
Lateral b147
Lateralization b230
Laterorotation b7200
Law e5952, e5902, e5901, e550
Laws e5952, e5502, e5501
Lead b122, d3500, d571
Leading b1343, d7700
Leaking e2600
Learning b144
Leave d2201
Leaving d8303, d8253, d8203, d8153,
    d2302 d845
Leg b7611, b7351, b7301, b760, s7501
Legal d7701, d760, d950, e5951, e550
Legally d7701
Legislation e5952, e5902, e5855, e5852,
    e5802, e5801, e5752, e5702, e5652,
    e5602, e5552, e5452, e5402, e5352,
    e5302, e5252, e5202, e5152, e5102,
    e550
Legislative e5951

Legs b7603, d4556, d4553, d4153, d4152,
    d4103, d4102, d435
Leisure d480, d920, d910, e5552, e5551,
    e5550
Lens b2150, s2204
Lenses e1251
Let d4403
Lethargy b1252
Letter d345, d2104, d2100, d170
Letters d1450, d1401, d1400, d166, d130
Lever e1550, e1500
Lie d410
Life b7610, b122, b117, e5152, e5151,
    e345, e340, e335, e325, e4
Lifestyle e580
Lift d4454, d440
Lifting d4556, d4400, d430
Lifts e1501
Ligaments s75023, s75013, s75003,
    s73023, s73013, s73003, s7703, s7602,
    s7403, s7203, s7105
Lighting d5700, e1602, e1601, e240
Limb b28015, b28014, b1801, b1474,
    b735, b730, d4554
Limbs b28015, b28014, b735, b730, d1201
Limit d240
Limited b1254
Limping b770
Lip s32041, s32040
Lips b5100, s3204, d3602, d1200
Liquid b5107, b5106, d1203, d5602
Liquids b510, d560, e1100
Listening d115
Litigation e5500
Liver s560
Living b520, d6102, d4600, d750, d640,
    d620, e215, e115
Lobe s11003, s11002, s11001, s11000
Lobes b164, s1100
Localization b230
Localized b280
Locate e1552, e1502
Locating d8450, e5250
Location b1141, b850, b230, d3352, d4,
    e540
Locations d460, e1552, e1502
Locomotion e2201, e2200
Lodging e525
Logic b1601

Logical b160
Longing b1302
Look b2152, d5702
Looking d2401, d110, d5, e590
Losing b2402
Lost b1440, d2401
Lotions d5200
Loud e2500
Loudness b230, b310
Love b152
Low b28013, b2400, b3101, e2500, e2251,
    e2250, e2151
Lower b28015, b4501, b4500, b735, b730,
    b440, s32041, s8104, s750, d7401,
    d4300, b4501, b4500, d5401, d5400,
    d435
Lowering d4305
Lubrication b640
Lumbar s76002
Lumbosacral s12002
Luminance b21022
Lungs b440, s4301
Lying d4555, d420, d415, d410
Lymph b4353, b4352
Lymphadenitis b435
Lymphatic b435, s4201, s4200
Lymphoedema b435

Maintain d6603
Maintaining b5501, b5452, b5451, b5450,
    b5108, b530, b420, d71041, d8301,
    d8251, d8201, d8151, d7504, d7503,
    d7502, d7501, d7500, d3551, d3550,
    d3504, d3503, d865, d845, d770, d760,
    d740, d720, d650, d161, d570, d410-
    d429, e5252, e5250, e5200
Majora s63031
Malabsorption b515
Manage d240, d230
Management b164, e5900
Managing d720, d640, d5301, d5300,
    d2203, d2202, d2200, d2103, d2102,
    d570, d250, d230
Manifestations b5550
Manipulate d446, d445, d150
Manipulating b510, d1310, d5301, d5300,
    d163, d155
Manipulation b5103, b172
Manipulations b1721

Mannerisms b765
Manners b340
Married d7701
Marriage d7701, d7602, e315, e310
Marriages d9102
Marrow b430, s4204
Master d830
Masticating b5102
Masturbation b640
Matching b21021
Mathematical b172, d172, d150
Mats e1450
Meal d6301, d6300, e5855, e5854, e5852,
    e5851
Meals d6604, d640, d630, d550
Meaning b1672, b1670, b122, d3352,
    d3351, d3152, d3151, d3150, d1702,
    d1700, d1661, d1402, d340, d330,
    d320, d145, d930, e145
Means d5102, d455, d360, d355, d350,
    d315
Meatus s2603
Mechanical d1701
Mechanisms b130, e5
Media e5350, e560
Medial b7200
Medical d6605, d830, d5702, e580, e355
Medication d6605, e1101
Medications d57020, d2305
Medicinal e1101
Meditating d163
Medium e1652, e1651, e1650
Medulla s11050
Meeting d9205, e5200
Melodiousness e2501
Melody b330, d3351, d332
Member d810
Members d660, d7, e5952, e425, e415,
    e410, e335, e325
Membership e555
Membrane s2500
Menarche b650
Mending d6500
Meninges s130
Menopause b6702, b650
Menorrhagia b650
Menstrual b6702, b6701, b650, d530
Menstruation b670, b660, b650,
    b555, d530

Mental b640, b230, b340, b330, b320, b310, d570, d210

Messages b1672, b1671, b1670

Metabolism b5, e2201

Metabolite b430

Metabolites b4302

Methodical b1262

Methods d6301, d6300, d1721, d510, e5602, e5601, e5352, e5351, e5350, e130

Midbrain s1101

Midline b7611

Migration e2150

Migratory d8500

Milestones b560

Milk b6603, d5602, d5601, e110

Mimicking d130

Mind b160, b152

Mineral b555, b545, b540

Minora s63032

Miscarriage b660

Missing b460, d2306

Misusing d571

Mixing d6301, d560

Mobility b7, d6504, d4, e5400, e5100, e1401, e350, e120, e115

Modified e11521, e1401

Modulating b3400

Modulation b3303

Moisture e2253, e2251

Moisturizing d5200

Molars b5102

Money d6201, d6200, d860, e165

Monitoring d845, e5901, e5854, e5851, e5801, e5751, e5701, e5651, e5601, e5551, e5501, e5451, e5401, e5351, e5301, e5251, e5201, e5151, e5101, e1

Monocular b210

Monoparesis b7401, b7351, b7301

Monoplegia b7401, b7351, b730

Monotone b3303

Moody b1263

Mopping d640

Moral e465

Morpheme d1451

Mosque d930

Mother d3503, d331

Motion b2401, e2254, e255

Motivation b130

Motor b765, b760, b755, b750, b147, d4751, d815, e1200

Motorized d6503, d475, d470, e1200

Mouth b510, b450, s320, d1200, d560, d550

Mouthing d1200

Move b5150, b735, b130, d4350, d4300, d470, d446, d445, e1201, e540

Movement b1472, b1344, b260, b235, b215, b176, b7, s7, d1314, d660

Movements b5100, b770, b765, b761, b760, b215, b176, b167, b147, d6601, d4554, d3350, d3150, d3100, d1551, e255

Moves b2152

Moving b5107, b5106, b5103, b2152, b1470, b1255, d8300, d8250, d8200, d8150, d7201, d6601, d1310, d4, e5402, e5401, e5400, e120

Mucus b450

Multicellular e2201, e2200

Multiple b2802, d1751, d2

Multiplication b1720, d1502

Muscle b4103, b780, b770, b765, b760, b455, b445, b440, b730-b749

Muscles b5352, b5250, b445, b410, b3100, b260, b215, b7, s75022, s75012, s75002, s73022, s73012, s73002, s7702, s7601, s7402, s7202, s7104, s4303, s2303

Muscular b5352

Musculoskeletal s770

Musical b3400, d3351, d3151, d920, e1401

Mutism b730

Mutual d7500, e5552, e5551, e5550, e320

Myalgia b280

Myasthenia b740

Myocarditis b410

Myopia b210

Myotonia b735

Nails b8, s830, d5100, d520

Nannies e340

Narcolepsy b134

Nasal s3300, s3102, s3101, d5205

Natural b1343, b1302, d7600, e5302, e2, e1

Nature b125, d7702, d7701, d1661, e2601, e2600, e2501, e2401

Naturopathic e1101

Nausea b535, b240
Neck b28010, s8100, s710
Need d5702, d5701, d177, d560, d550, d530
Needing b5350
Needs b130, d870, d570, e5
Negativism b147
Negotiating d6200
Neighbourhood d6601, d4602
Neighbours d750, e425, e325
Nerve b2804, b2803
Nerves s1201, s1106
Neural e1151
Neuromusculoskeletal b215, b176, b7
Newspapers d166, e560
Nieces e315
Nipple b55501, s6302
Nodding b7653
Nodes b435, s4201
Noises d160, e2501
Non-rapid eye movement b1344
Non-verbal b1471, d335, d315
Nose s310, d1202, d520
Notation d3351
Notations d3151
Notes b340
Notice d845
Novelty b126, d2500
Noxious b750, b270
NREM b1344
Nuclear d760
Number b6201, b4400, b4100, d6301, d6300, d172, e2151, e2150
Numbers b1721, b1720, d172, d150, e5855, e5854, e5852, e5851
Numbness b2702, b265
Numeracy d1720, d1501
Numerals d1500
Nurses e355
Nurture d7600
Nurturing e3
Nutrients b520, b515
Nutrition d660
Nutritious d5701
Nystagmus b215

Obesity b530
Obeying d7601

Objects b21003, b21002, b21001, b21000, b1640, b1565, b1250, b1143, b163, d1202, d1201, d1200, d9203, d2500, d2102, d134, d133, d131, d880, d6, d4, e1553, e11521, e11520, e510, e165
Oblongata s11050
Observation d8801
Obsession b1603
Obsessions b160
Obstacles d455, d450
Obstruction b610, b515, b440
Obtain b1670
Obtaining d8451, d8302, d8252, d8202, d8152, d6201, d6200, d166, d132
Occasion d6301
Occipital s11003
Occupation d850, d845
Occupational e5900, e355
Occupations e5902, e5901
Occupying d880
Occurrences b6500
Occurring e2150, e230
Occurs b6201
Ocular b1561, s2303
Oculomotor b176
Odour b830, e2601, e2600
Odours b255
Oesophageal b5105
Oesophagus b5107, b5106, b5105, s520
Olfactory b255, b156
Oligozoospermia b660
Oliguria b610
Oneself b2401, b1800, b1644, b1565, d7204, d7200, d4451, d4450, d3500, d630, d465, d455, d450, d420, d410, d2200, d880, d5
Onset b6503, b5550, b134
Open d4501, e520, e515
Opening d560, d550
Openness b126
Operating e5401
Operation d150, e5952
Operations b172, d1720, d150
Opinion b1645, d7103
Opinions e460, e455, e450, e445, e440, e435, e430, e425, e420, e415, e410
Opportunities d940
Oppositional b1261

Optical e1250
Optimal b54501, b5501, b1343
Optimism b126
Options b1645, d177, d175
Oral b5105, s3301, d330
Order b16703, b16702, d4455, d4300,
    d870, d650, d5101, d5100, d145,
    d230, e575
Ordering b1642, d1501
Ordinating b176
Organize e5951
Organisms e2201, e2200
Organization b1472, b1103, b164,
    b163, e5101
Organizational e325, e5
Organizations d930, d910
Orgasm b6700, b640
Orgasmic b640
Orientation b156, b147, b144, b114, b110
Orography e210
Orthoses d6504
Orthosis d5201
Orthotic e1151
Ossicles s2502
Outdoor d650, e5400, e260, e160, e155,
    e150, e120, e115
Outgoing b1260
Outside d6505, d4500, d660, d460, d9,
    e1552, e1502, e360, e260, e120
Ovaries s6300
Overweight b530
Ownership d6100
Owning d8500
Oxygen b5400, b430
Ozone e2601

Pacing d210
Pain b840, b780, b670, b650, b630, b535,
    b460, b167
Painful b7501, b5352, b2703
Painting d3352, d650
Palate s3202
Palpitation b460
Pancreas s550
Pants d540
Paradoxical b440
Paraesethesia b2702
Paraesthesia b265
Paraffin e240
Parallel d8802

Paralysis b7402, b7356, b730, b515
Parameters b560
Paramyotonia b735
Paraparesis b7401, b7353, b7303
Paraplegia b7401, b7353, b730
Paraplegic b770
Parasympathetic s150
Parathyroid s5802
Parent d760
Parental d7600
Parents d7602, d7601, d810, e310, d240
Paresis b7402, b7356, b730
Parietal s11002
Parkinson b7356
Parks d9103, e520, e160
Participants d2205, e320
Participating d8450, d3504
Partner d7702
Partners d770, e310
Passage b5105, b1802, b310
Passages d330
Passenger d470
Passing b5152
Pastimes d9204
Patellar b750
Paths e5402, e5401, e5400
Pathways e1601, e1600
Pattern b770, b765, b760, d2504, d2503,
    d2502, e2501, e215
Patterns b770, b3303, b3301, b125, d3100
Pay d855
Paying d6200
Pedals d435
Pedestrian e5200
Peeling d6301
Peers d8301, d8251, d8201, d8151, d750,
    e425, e325
Pelvic b28012, s8103, s740, s620
Pelvis b720
Penal e5500
Pencil d4400, d1450
Penile b640
Penis b55502, s6305
Pension e5700
Pensions e5702, e5701
People b1403
Perception b156
Perceptual b230, b210, b167, b160, b156,
    b144, b140
Perform d1720, d150

Performance b640, e1401, e340
Period b740, b530, b140, d7200, d4155
Periodic b134, e5800
Periodicity b4401
Peripheral b210, d1450
Peristalsis b515
Permit b1403, b1402, b1401
Permitting b1441
Perserveration b765
Perseveration b7653, b1601, b147
Persistence b750, b125
Persistent b130
Person b4551, b1603, b114
Personal b126, b125, b122, e5400,
    e575, e440, e350, e340, e310, e120,
    e115, e110
Personality b152, b130, b126, b125
Persons b1255, d7106, d1630, d1600,
    d8802, d740, d350, d137, d134, d133,
    d132, d110, d940, d250, e5402, e5401,
    e5400, e5250, e590, e3
Pet d4403, d4302
Pets d650, d2204, e350
Pharmacologically b110
Pharyngeal b5105
Pharynx b5105, s330
Phase b640
Phases b6701
Phenomenon e250
Philosophies e465
Philtrum s3205
Phonation b310
Phonemes b320
Phonetic d1660
Photophobia b21020
Photosensitivity b810
Photosynthetic e2201, e2200
Phrases d330, d145, d140, d134, d133
Physical b1144, b810, b640, b455, b134
Physicians d9101
Physiotherapists e355
Picking d440
Pictograms d3152
Piercing b5101
Pigmentation b860, b850, b810
Pitch b3400, b3303, b230, b310
Pitches b1560
Pituitary s5800

Place b114, d8450, d6601, d650, d640,
    d620, d610, d5301, d5300, d2205,
    d2105, d2101, d4, e3
Placement e5900
Places d1630, d9205, d460, e1552, e1502
Placing b7603
Plan d230
Planning b164, d6506, d6406, d630,
    d2205, d530, e5402, e520, e515, e160
Plans b164, d230
Planting d6505
Plants d650, e220
Play e1152, e140, e3
Playground e11521
Playing d3504, d720, d2105, d2103,
    d2101, d163, d155, d131, d110, d920
Playmates d750
Pleasure d920
Point d2402
Pointing d3350
Points d2402
Police e5452, e5451, e5450
Policy e5952, e5201
Polishing d6500, d5204, d5203
Political d325, d950, d940, d920, d910,
    e595, e4
Pollution e235
Polymenorrhoea b650
Polyuria b620
Pondering d163
Pons s11051
Population e5300, e220, e215
Porch d4600
Portability e5802, e5801
Portable e1550, e1500
Position b1565, b755, b260, b235, b180,
    d7402, d7401, d7400, d7203, d5700,
    d5301, d5300, e2451
Positions d7401, d7400, d410, e5950,
    e435, e430, e335, e330
Possession b110
Postnatal b7611
Postural b755, b420
Posture d4101
Postures d3350, d3150
Posturing b147
Potassium b545
Potential b280, d175

Pouring d560

Power b770, b760, b740, b735, b730, d7400, d930, e5951, e2200, e1550, e1500, e330

Powered d475, d470, e1200

Practice e145

Practices d930, d570 e5302

Practising d135

Prayer e1450

Prayers d4152, d4102

Praying d930

Precipitation e225

Predictability b125

Predictable b1253, e2255, e245

Preference b1474, b1473

Pregnancy b660

Pregnant b6601

Premature b660, b640

Premenstrual b650

Preparation b6700, d6301, d6300, d840, d825, d815, e5900

Preparatory b640

Prepare d6604, d6302, d815

Preparing d845, d640, d630, d2305, d2204, d2203, d2202, d2200, d2103, d2102, d2101, d2100

Preschool d816, d815, e5853, e5850

Presence b230, b210, d8802

Presenting d6301

Press e5602, e5601, e5600

Pressure b420, b415, b410, b270, b240, b220, b160, d2401, e225

Prestige d7402, d7401, d7400

Pretence d1314

Pretend d131

Pretending d1314, d163

Prevent d5702

Preventing e580, e1

Prevention e5800

Priaprism b640

Primary b5550, b650, b530, s32000, d820, e5853, e5850, e5800, e340

Principles d172, e5150

Private d4602, d4601, d870, d470, e340, e155

Privileges d820, d950

Problems e580

Procedure d331

Procedures d1721, d230

Proceeding b1641

Process b5403, b5402, b5401, b1602, b1601, b1600 d8302, d8252, d8202, d8152, d1721, d1720, d1700, d1660

Processes b172, b152, e1301

Processing b1442

Procreation b670, b660, b650, b640

Procuring d620

Producing b1470, b1262, b450, b3, d6500, d172, d170, d3, e2200

Production b6603, b5104, b1672, b555, b540, b515, b340, b330, b320, b310, b4, e565, e510

Products e5400, e5200, e510, e1

Profession d850, d845, d825

Professional d7201, d7200, d830, d5702, d910, e5900, e5853, e5850

Professionals d57021, d740, e455, e450, e360, e355, e340

Professions d750

Programme d8303, d8302, d8301, d8253, d8252, d8251, d8250, d8203, d8202, d8201, d8200, d8153, d8152, d8151, d8150

Programme d825, d820, e5852, e5752

Programmes d840, d830, d920

Progressing d8302, d8252, d8202, d8152

Promote d815

Promoting e580

Promotion d8451, e5800, e590

Prone d4550, d4150

Pronunciation d140

Propel d4454, d4351

Propelling d4556, d4555, d4554

Proper b1471, d1701, d650, d5301, d5300, d2402

Properties b126, b125, d137

Property d865, e545, e165

Proprioceptive b260

Prosody b330

Prostate s6306

Prostheses d6504, e1251, e1151

Prosthesis d5201

Prosthetic e1151

Prosthetists e355

Prostrate d4150, d4100

Protecting b810

Protection b860, b850, b830, b435, e1451, e545, e530, e3

Protective b2151, b830, b820, b810
Protein b540
Proteins b540
Protraction b7200
Provide b1603, e260, e250, e240
Provider e57501
Providers d7201, d740, e575, e440, e360,
    e355, e345, e340, e310
Provides e3
Providing d7600, d7103, e5600, e5550,
    e5500, e5250, e580, e575, e570
Proving d163
Provision d6606, e5802, e5801, e5751,
    e5550, e5452, e5451, e5402, e5352,
    e5302, e5301, e560, e525
Psychic b126
Psychological d240, e5802, e5801, e5800,
    e350
Psychomotor b176, b160, b147, b140,
    b134, b130, b126, b125
Psychosocial b122
Ptosis b215
Pubertal b5550
Puberty b5550
Pubic b55500, s8403
Public d4602, d4601, d3151, d9205,
    d9103, d870, d470, d2304, e340,
    e150, e5
Pulling d5401, d445
Pulmonary b440, b415, b410
Pumping b410
Punctuation d1701
Pupil b2150
Pupillar b2150
Pupillary b215
Purchase d860, d730
Purchasing d177
Purpose b122, d7503, d8803, d166, d930
Purposeful b176, d1550, d880,
    d110-d129
Purposive b765
Pursue e325
Pursuit e555
Pushing d445, d435
Pyloric b5106

Quadriceps b750
Quadriplegia b730
Qualities b1640, b250, b310

Quality b7610, b860, b810, b265, b230,
    b210, b147, b134, b110, b310, d6200,
    d1601, b7611
Quantity b6502, d1601, d1370
Question d1750
Questions d3500, d3102, d175
Queue d4154
Quitting d8452
Quivering e255

Radiating b2804, b2803
Radiation b810, e240
Rain e2601, e2253
Raising d430
Ramps e1602, e1550, e1500
Rapid eye movement b1344
Rate b5105, b540, b440, b410, b3302,
    e1151
Reaching b6402, d7106, d4105, d445
React b126, b125
Reacting d7104
Reaction b755
Reactions b755, b435
Read d9202, d166, d140
Readiness d815
Reading d2104, d2100, d166, d920
Realizing d315
Reasoning b163
Reattaching d6500
Recalling b144
Receive d3350, e1251
Receiving b1520, d3, e125
Receptive b167
Reciprocal b122
Recitation d135
Reciting d2401
Recognize d1500, d1400
Recognizing b167, b156, d1660, d140
Record d170
Recreation d480, d920, d910, e5550,
    e1152, e325, e140
Recreational d6504, d920, e5552, e5551,
    e5200, e140
Rectum b5250
Recurrent b5106
Recurring b1302
Reducing b5151
Reduction b440
Reemployment e5900

Reflex b755, b750, b620, b215
Reflux b5106
Refocusing b1401
Refrigerating d6404
Regard d1312, d1311
Region b28012, b2804, s8103, s8101,
 s8100, s740, s720, s710, e5855, e5854,
 e5852, e5851
Registering b144
Registration e5952
Regular d6605, e2255, e255, e245
Regulate b1470, b1304, e5
Regulating b5500, b1103, d720, d530
Regulation b1103, b555, b550, b545,
 b540, b152, e5952, e5351, e1501
Regulations e5
Regurgitating b5107
Regurgitation b510
Rehabilitation e580
Rehearsing d135
Rehydration b5450
Rejecting b5153
Relating b6501, b239, b210, d7600, d1313,
 d1312, d1311, d740, d730, e555
Relation b1565, b114, e2451
Relations d7402, d7401, d7400, d660,
 e5900
Relationship b1144, b126, b125, d8500,
 d7702, d7701, d7700, d7603, d7602,
 d7200, e345, e310
Relationships b122, d6603, d7, e5552,
 e5551, e4, e3
Relative b1565, b260, d7402, d7401,
 d7400, d6605
Relatives d9205, d7
Relaxation b7651, b6403, b1343, d920
Releasing d440
Relief e210
Religion d950, d930, d920, d910, e145
Religious d9102, d855, d325, d930, e5552,
 e5551, e5550, e5502, e5501, e1451,
 e335, e330, e325, e4
REM b1344
Remaining d415
Remembering b144
Removing d5200, d540
Remuneration d855
Remunerative d855, d850, d660, d650,
 d920, d910, e5902, e5901

Renal b610
Renting d610
Repair b830, b820, b810, d6501, e5300
Repairing b820, d6
Repeating d135, d130
Repertoire b7611, b7610
Repetition b3300
Repetitive b7652, b3301
Replacement e5700
Reporting e5602, e5601, e5600
Representation b1801, b163, e5500
Representations d3152
Requirement d8302, d8252, d8202, d8152
Requirements d8301, d8251, d8151, d820,
 d2400, d230, e5352
Residence d4601, d4600, d750
Residential e5802, e5801, e5800, e5300,
 e5152, e5151, e5150
Resist b1304
Resistance b735
Resistant b1250
Resolution b6700, b640
Resolving d175
Resources d870, e5900
Respect d710
Respiration b4, s430
Respiratory b3100
Respite e575
Respond d5702
Responding d710, d310, d2501, d2300
Response b4202, b1470, b435, d1550,
 d331, d2304, d250, e2201
Responses b435, b125, d7106
Responsibilities d820, d240, e330
Responsivity b125
Rest b5400, b1343
Resting b735
Restlessness b1470
Restricted b1260, d4600, e2201
Retardation b1470, b117
Retention b620, b545
Retina s2203
Retinacula s7703
Retraction b7200
Retreating b1255
Retrieving b144, d3501
Retrograde b650
Returning d2302
Reverse b5107, b5106

Reversibility d1371
Rhyme d135
Rhythm b1340, b440, b410, b340, b330
Rice d6300
Riding d4700, d480, d920
Right b21003, b21001, b7352, b7302,
    b2303, b760, d2402, d950, d940
Rights d950, d940, e165
Ringing b240, e250
Rise b4200
Rising d4555
Risks d5702, d571
Rites d9102
Rituals e465
Rocking b7653
Role d7203, d950
Roles e330
Rolling d455, d410
Romantic d7201, d7200, d770
Room d4600, d610, d430, d2105, d2101
Rooms d6102, d4500, d650, d640, d460
Rooting b7502
Rotate d4453
Rotating b2401
Routine d230
Routing e155, e150
Rubs d315
Rules d1551, d9200, d720, d2103,
    d940, e465
Ruminating b5108
Rumination b1603
Run d7503, d950
Running b770, d8500, d2306, d571,
    d560, d4
Rushing b2400

Saccadic b2152
Sacral s76003
Sadness b152
Safe d570
Safeguarding e545
Safety d571, e5900, e5401, e5302, e5301,
    e5152, e5151, e1553, e1503
Saliva b5104
Salivary s510
Salivation b510
Salting d6404
Sanitation e530
Satiation d5602, d5601
Satisfaction b6403, d7101

Satisfy b130
Sauntering d450
Saving d860
Scab b820
Scalp d520
Scampering d455
Scapula b720
Scarring b820
School d8253, d6601, d4303, d3504,
    d2304, d2302, d2201, d2105, d2101,
    d835, d830, d820, d815, d415, e5855,
    e5854, e5853, e5852, e5851, e5850,
    e5802, e5801, e5800, e3
Schooling d810
Schools d830, e5855, e5854, e5852, e5851,
    e1500
Sclera s2200
Scooters d6504, e1201
Scooting d455
Scotoma b210
Scratching b860
Screaming b340
Scripture d325
Scrotum b55502, s6304
Search d950, e5900
Seat d4200, d4153, d4151
Seating e1501
Sebaceous s8201
Secondary b5550, b650, b530, d820,
    e5853, e5850
Secretion b830
Securing d2205
Security d870, e5902, e5901, e5401, e575,
    e570, e565
Seeing b2, d110, b156
Seek d9200, d2103
Seeking b126, d850, d845, d5702, e590
Seen b2101
Seize d4401
Seizure d950
Selecting d630, d620, d5701, d177
Selective b144, b134
Self b1266, b180, b122, b114, d870, d850,
    d660, d940, d930, d5, e575
Semantic b1672, b1441
Semicircular s2602
Send e1251
Sensation b840, b780, b670, b650, b535,
    b460

Sensations b2703, b840, b780, b670, b650,
    b640, b630, b620, b535, b525, b515,
    b510, b280, b260, b240, b220,
    b450-b469
Sense b235, d115, d110
Senses b2, d120
Sensing b270, b265, b260, b255, b250,
    b230, b210, d120
Sensitive b270
Sensitivity b2703, b2702, b2701, b2700,
    b2102
Sensitization b4351, b4350
Sensory b167, b156, d110-d129
Sentences d3102, d1702, d134, d133
Sentience b1102
Separate d230
Separating b21022
Separation b2301
Septa s7703
Septum s3101
Sequence b1642, b1471, d2306, d2304,
    d2105, d2101, d1551, d540, d332,
    d220, d135
Sequences b1472
Sequencing b176, b147
Sequentially d2203, d2202, d2201, d2200
Seriation d1371
Serve e1652, e1651, e1650
Served b2804, b2803, d550
Service d7201, d910, d840, d740
Services d860, d815, d650, d640, d630,
    d620, d610, e1652, e1651, e1650, e340,
    e325, e5
Serving d630
Settling e5500
Severe e230
Sewing d6500
Sex d570
Sexual b555, b6, d770, d5702
Shaft s63051
Shakiness b7651
Shaking b270, d335, e255
Shape b2150, b1561, b210
Shaping d3551, d3550, d3504, d3503,
    d3501
Share d7504, e325, e215
Shares d7602
Sharing b140, e345
Shaving d5202

Shelter e5252
Sheltering e5252, e5251
Shelters e525
Shifting b1643, b140, d410
Shoe d2104, d2100
Shop d8500, d6200, d4503
Shopping d620, d2201, e575
Short b144, d8500, d7200, d4602, d450,
    e5800
Shortages e5302
Shortness b460
Shoulder b28016, b715, b710, s8101, s720
Shoulders d5401, d5400, d430
Shower d5101
Showering d510
Showing d8450, d710
Shuffling d455
Shy b1260
Sibling d760
Siblings e310
Sick d6600
Side b2303, b735, b730, d4150, d410
Sideways d450
Sight b1565
Sign b167, d3501, d355, d340, d320
Signage e1603, e1552, e1502
Signalling e1251
Signals e1553, e1503
Signed b1671, d350
Signing d134
Signposting e1602, e1601, e1600
Signs b167, d7104, d1330, d150
Silence d1661, d1660
Simple b760, b172, d3101, d1720, d1550,
    d860, d630, d250, d240, d230, d220,
    d210, d175, d150, d131
Singing b340, d9202, d332
Sitting d4555, d420, d415, d410
Situation b1520
Situations b126, e325
Sketching d3352
Skill d155, e130
Skills b122, d1721, d1720, d1702, d1700,
    d1660, d1502, d1501, d1500, d1452,
    d1451, d1450, d1402, d1401, d1400,
    d815, d810, d220, d210, d155, d132,
    e1652, e585
Skin b2804, b2803, b2702, b8, s8, d520
Skipping d455

Skirts d540

Sleep b7650, b140, b134, b130, b110

Sleeping b134

Sleet e2253

Slicing d6301

Sliding d420

Slippery d4154

Slope d4154

Sloping d4502

Slow b4400, b4100

Smell b255, e2601, e2600

Smelling b255, d120

Smells b1562, b255, e2601

Smiling d3350

Smoke e2601, e2600

Smooth b5352, b1564, b3300

Sneezing b450

Snow d4502, e2253

Soap d5101, d5100

Soccer d9201

Sociable b1260

Social b122

Socializing d920

Society d5404, e460, e330, e5

Socket s210

Sodium b545

Software e1351, e1300, e1251

Solids b510

Solitary d8800, d2102

Solution b1646, d175

Solutions d175

Solve d172

Solvents e1553

Solving b1646, b1643, d220, d210

Somatization b1602

Somersaulting d455

Songs d332

Sorrow b152

Sorting d2102

Sought d8500

Sound b3100, b230, d1401, d331, d130,
    e1250, e250

Sounding d140

Sounds b1560, b230, b3, d331, d145,
    e2500

Source b230, e2400

Sources d870, e5951

Space b114, d2203, d2202, d2200, d720,
    d465, d210, d6, e520, e515, e160

Spaces d9103, e5200

Span b144, b122, b117

Spasm b780, b535, b440

Spasmodic b5352

Spastic b770, b320

Spasticity b735

Speaking b1470, d6602, d3501, d330

Spectrum b1522

Speculating d163

Speech b230, b176, b167, b3, s3, d950,
    d331, e355

Speed b5105, b2352, b1600, b1470, b330

Spelling d1701, d145

Sphincter b525

Spinal s120

Spirit e1450

Spiritual d930

Spirituality d930, d920, d910, e145

Spitting b510

Spleen b430, s4203

Spoken b2304, b167, d1452, d355, d350,
    d330, d310

Spontaneity b1470

Spontaneous b7653, b761, b660, d9200

Sport e1152, e140

Sporting d2205, d110, e5550, e140

Sports d2205, d920, e1401

Spousal d770

Spouse d7702, d7701

Spouses e310

Spring d560, e2255

Squatting d415, d410

Stabbing b280

Stability b715, b710, b126

Stable b1253, b1103

Stage d8300, d8250, d8200

Stages b640, d820

Stagnant b1264

Stairs d4551, e2401

Stamina b1300, b455

Stammering b330

Standing d415, d410, d950

Starting d7200, d355, d350

State b1342, b1340, b110, d1632, e5

States b110

Statesthesia b260

Stationary e1550, e1500

Staying d415

Stem s1105

Stenosis b5106
Step d760, d450
Steps d4552, d4551, d2203, d2103
Stereotypes b147
Stereotypic b3301
Stereotypies b765
Sterility b660
Sticks d4402
Stiff b770
Stiffness b780
Stimulation e1151
Stimuli b1402, b755, b750, b270, b265,
    b210, b156, d160, d120, d115, d110,
    e2201
Stimulus b270, b140
Stirring d6301, d6300, d560
Stomach b28012, b5107, b5106, b5105,
    b535, b515, s530, d4107
Stool b525
Stop d4455
Store b1440
Storing b144, d640, d620
Story d330, d115
Straight d4153
Strain b220
Strangers d355, d350, e445, e345
Strategies b1643, d1721, d1720, d1702,
    d1700, d1660
Stray b21023
Street d9103, d465, d460, d455, e1602,
    e1601
Stress b620, b3301, d2
Stretch b750
Stretching b7500
String d4450
Strolling d450
Structural b715, d1660
Structures b730, b220, b215, e5951, e5950
Student d8301, d8251, d8201, d8151,
    d835
Students d820, d750, e335
Study d830
Studying d820
Stupor b110
Stuttering b330
Styling d5202
Subcomponents b1471
Subfertility b660
Subjective b1802

Subjects d820
Subordinate e435, e335
Subordinates d740
Subsidies e5855, e5854, e5852, e5851
Substance b43500, e110
Substances b435, b130, d5101, d5100,
    e110
Substitute e345, e330
Substituting d1314
Subtraction b172, d150
Suburban e520, e160
Subway d470
Sucking b510, d1203
Suckle d5602, d5601
Suction b5100
Sufficiency d870
Suitable b5153, e590
Supervising d6201, d6200, d855, d850
Supervisors e330
Supine d4150
Supplements e1100
Supply b4103, e5302
Supplying e5300
Support d4554, e590, e580, e575,
    e570, e165
Supporting b755, d4155
Supportive b760
Supports d2305
Surface d4305, d465, d450, d420, e5351,
    e5350
Surfaces b265, d4551, d4154, d640, d450,
    e1552, e1502
Surrounding b3100, e2252
Surroundings b114, e2401
Susceptibility b4552
Sustain b1342
Sustaining b3400, b740, b140, d355, d350,
    d210, d161
Sutures s71000
Swabbing d6402
Swallowing b510
Swaying b2401
Sweat b830, s8200
Sweating b830
Sweeping d640
Swim d465
Swimming d455
Swings e11520
Switches e1351, e1151

Symbol d1451, d1450
Symbolic b1672, d3351, d131, e145
Symbolically d1313
Symbols b172, b167, d1500, d170, d166,
    d145, d140, d135, d134, d133, d3
Sympathetic s140
Sympathy d7100
Synagogue d930
Syntax d1332
Synthesis b2301
System b1441, b3100, b540-b569, b510-
    b539, b4, s630, s610, s430, s420, s410,
    s1, e5952, e5855, e5852, e5802, e5801,
    e565, e360, e355, e1
Systematically d2401
Systematizing b1641
Systems d3351, e465
Systolic b4201, b4200

Tachycardia b410
Tachylalia b330
Tachypnoea b4400
Tactile b156
Talking d331
Tap d560
Tapping b1470
Target b2152
Tarsal b720
Tasks b163, e1351
Taste b250, d1203
Tastes b1563
Tasting b2, d120
Tax e570
Taxi d470
Taxonomic b126, b125, d8251, d8151,
    d820, d740, e360, e345, e330
Tear b2153
Tearing b5101
Technologies e160, e125, e120, e115
Technology d2305, e5802, e5801, e5400,
    e5100
Teeth b5103, b5102, b5101, s3200, d4453,
    d520
Telecommunication d360, e5351
Telephone d360, e5352, e5351, e5350,
    e1250
Teletext e5350
Teletype e5350
Television e1250, e560

Telex d3600
Telling d330
Temperament b152, b130, b126,
    b125
Temperature b5400, b550, b270, b265,
    e1501, e225
Temple d930
Temples e1451
Temporal s11001, e245
Tension b1470, b735, b650, b152
Terminate d6603
Terminating b3400, d8303, d8253, d8203,
    d8153, d3551, d3550, d3504, d3503,
    d845, d720
Termination d3502
Test d1632
Testes b55502, s6304
Tetraparesis b7402, b7354, b7304
Tetraplegia b7402, b7354, b7304
Text d166
Texts d1402
Texture b1564, b265, d5200
Textures d120
Therapists e355
Thermoregulatory b555, b550, b540
Thigh s7500
Thin b1801
Thinking b1603, b1602, b1601, b1600,
    b164, d1
Thinning b810
Thoracic b445, s76001, s12001,
    s4302
Thought b172, b167, b164, b160, b144,
    b117, d1632
Thoughts d350
Threatening b755
Threats b810
Thresholds e1550, e1500
Thromboembolism b415
Throwing d445
Thumb d440
Thumping e250
Thymus s4202
Thyroid s5801
Tics b765
Tidying d640
Tightness b780, b460
Tilting d4105, b2401
Timbre e250

Time b6501, b1470, b1344, b1340, b740, b180, b164, b140, b114, d7200, d4155, d4154, d4153, d4152, d4150, d2205, d2203, d2202, d2200, d855, d850, d240, d230, d210, d161, e245
Timid b1266
Tingling b2702, b840, b265
Tinnitus b240
Tired b220, d315
Toe b1470, s8301, d520
Toenails d5204
Toes s75021, d5204, d446
Toilet d4200
Toileting d6600, d530, d520, d510
Toilets d6402, d4101
Tolerance b5501, b740, b515, b4, d710
Tone b770, b740, b735, b730, e250
Tones b1560, d332
Tongue b5103, b5100, b1563, s3203
Tool d4401, d1551
Tools d6504, d6502, d6501, d620, d155, e1350, e1150
Torso d4105
Torticollis b7350
Tossing d4454
Touch b1564, b270, b265, d4452, d1600
Touching b265, d120
Towel d510
Towels d5302
Tower d2104, d2100
Town b1141, d7201, d4501, d9103, d460
Toxic e2601, e235
Toy b1403, d4451, d1313, d1310, d430
Toys d1313, d1312, d1311, d9203, d2105, d2101, d155, d880, e11521, e11520, e1300
Trachea s4300
Track d2401
Tracking b215, d110
Tract b5352, b515
Trade d850, d845, d825, e5902, e5901
Trading d865
Traffic d4503, d3151, d571, d240
Train d4502, d2306, d470
Trainers e1251
Training d840, d825, e5100, e585
Trance b110
Transaction d865, d860
Transactions d8
Transfer e1201

Transferring d4
Transforming d6301, d6300
Transition b1341
Transitioning d8300, d8250, d8200
Transitions d2304
Translating b1721
Transmission e1250, e535
Transmitting e5350
Transport b4352, b515, d2304, e5400, e575, e340
Transportation b4501, d2205, d920, d4, e5200, e5100, e540, e530, e350, e120, e115
Transporting b515, b450, b415, d4304, d4303, d4302, d4301, d620
Transpose d1452, d1451
Travelling d920, d480, d475
Treating e580
Tremor b7651
Tremors b765
Tricycle d4750
Tricycles e1200
Trimming d5204, d5203, d5202
Trunk b28013, b735, b730, s8105, s760
Trust e320
Trustees e330
Trustworthiness b126, e4
Trying b735
Tubes s63012
Tunnel b210
Turning d4107, d445, d2402
Twisting d445
Tying d4402
Tympanic s2500
Type d815
Types d163, e5700, e5401
Typewriters d3601

Ulcers b810
Uncomfortable b2703
Unconscious b1301
Uncontrolled e2600
Undergarments d540
Understand b122, b117, d137
Understanding b1644, d7102, d3152, d325, d310, d140
Undertake d177
Undertaking d177, d161, d230, d220, d210
Underweight b530

Undigested b525
Unemployed e590
Unemployment e5752, e5751, e5750, e570
UNESCO e585
Uneven d4502
Unfamiliar e345
Unfriendly b1261
Unintentional b765
Uninterrupted b3300
Union e5950
Unions e5902, e5901
Unique d166, e145
Unit e2151
United d940, e5950
Units e1351, e1151
Universal d940
Universality e5802, e5801
Universities d830
Unmarried d7701
Unorganized d9200
Unpleasant b280
Unpredictable b1253
Unproven d1632
Unreasonable d950
Unrelated e345
Unreliable b1262
Unstable b715
Unstructured d9200, e1152
Unsuitable b5153
Unsupported d4153, d4103
Upper b28014, b4501, b4500, b440, s32040, s8102, s730, d5401, d5400
Ureteric b610
Ureters b6101, s6101
Urethra s6103
Urge b1303, b620
Urgency b620
Urges b1304
Urinary b670, b610-b639, s610
Urination b6, d530
Urine b630, b620, b610
Utensils d4453, d1550, d640, d620, e1150
Uterus s6301
Utilities d620, e5652, e5651, e5650, e545, e530
Utilization b5452, b5451

Vacuum d640
Vagina s6303

Vaginal b640, s63033
Vaginismus b640
Valuables e165
Valves b415, b410
Vans e1201, e1200
Variation b3400, e2255, e2150
Varicose b415
Variety e5802, e5801, e5800, e5352, e5351, e5350
Various b310, b117, d5401, d5400, d4, e2200, e5
Vascular b4352
Vasomotor b415
Vegetable d6201
Vegetative b110
Vehicle d4502, d475, d470, d240
Vehicles d4700, d4503, d650, d475, e5401, e1201, e1200,
Vehicular e5200
Veins b415, s4102
Venous b4152
Ventricles s41001
Ventricular b410
Ventures e5650
Verbal d3503, d720
Vertebral b710, s7600
Vertigo b240
Vessel b420, b415, b410
Vessels b4, s4200
Vestibular b260, b156, b230-b249, s2601
Vibration b270, e255
Vigour b1300
Violent e230
Virtue d940
Visible e240
Vision e1251
Visit d7201
Visiting d9205
Visual b2152, b210, b156, d110, e2401
Visually b7602, d110
Visuospatial b156
Vitae d845
Vitamin e1100
Vitreous s2205
Vocal b3400, b765, s3400, d3503
Vocalizing d3501, d331
Vocalization b340
Vocalizations b3401, b3400
Vocational d840, d825, e5900, e585

Voice b167, d3100, d1600, d115, e1351, e1251, e1151
Voiding b6200, b630
Volitional b1603
Volume b4402, b4103, e250
Voluntary b5253, b770, b765, b760, b710, b215, e340, e5
Volunteer d855
Vomit b5350, b5108, b2403
Vomiting b510
Vote d950
Voting e595

Waiting d2401
Wakeful b110
Wakefulness b1341, b1103, b1101
Walker d465
Walkers d6504
Walking b770, d4, e1201
Walls d640, e2200
Want e1552, e1502
Wanting b2403
Warm d570
Warmth d710
Warning d315
Wash d4453
Washing d6502, d640, d5
Washroom e1551, e1501
Waste b5250, d530
Wastes b525
Wasting b530
Water b555, b545, b540, d6201, d4554, d4553, d4305, d4304, d2204, d560, d510, e5402, e5401, e5400, e1200, e530, e235, e210
Watering d650
Watery b525
Wave d1550, e2501
Wavelength e2501
Way b126, b125, d2304, e1552, e1502
Ways d4503, d465, d560, d550
Weakness b730
Weapons e1553
Weather d3503, e230, e225
Web e5602, e5601, e5600
Webbing b21023

Weight b7603, b540, b530, b520, d4155, d4106
Welfare e5702, e5701, e5700
Well-being e5800
Wheelchair d4200, d465
Wheelchairs d6504, e1201
Wheezing b460
Whistling b450, e250
Wife d770
Wiggling b7653
Wildlife e5202, e5201, e160
Wincing d3350
Wind e225
Windows d6402
Withdrawal b750
Withdrawing b1255
Wood d1314, d9203
Word b1721
Words b3300, d3102, d3101, d1702, d1700, d1660, d330, d172, d163, d145, d140, d134, d133
Work d7201, d6501, d2304, d2302, d2204, d920, d415, d8, e5802, e5801, e5800, e590, e135, e3
Workers d855, d850, d750, e360, e355, e345, e335
Working b1262, d9203, d8500, d6406, d6302, d855, d820, d650, e360, e355
Workplaces e1500
World e5602, e5601, e5600, e465, e260, e250, e240
Worried b1263
Wringing b1470
Wrist b710, s73011
Write d170, d155, d145
Writhing b7610
Writing d6602, d2104, d2100, d170, d155, d145, d3, e1552, e1502

Xerophthalmia b215

Yawning b450
Yelling e250
Young d7601

Zinc b545